Historical Foundations of Liver Surgery

Thomas S. Helling • Daniel Azoulay

Historical Foundations of Liver Surgery

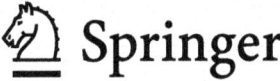 Springer

Thomas S. Helling
University of Mississippi Medical Center
Jackson, MS
USA

Daniel Azoulay
Centre Hépato-Biliaire
Hôpital Universitaire Paul Brousse
Villejuif
France

ISBN 978-3-030-47094-4   ISBN 978-3-030-47095-1   (eBook)
https://doi.org/10.1007/978-3-030-47095-1

This Springer imprint is published by the registered company Springer Nature Switzerland AG
The registered company address is: Gewerbestrasse 11, 6330 Cham, Switzerland

For Tom

Preface

There have been remarkable advances in the field of liver surgery over the past one hundred years. What had once been feared as an unforgiving and treacherous domain has now been almost routinely assailed, prodded, sliced, gouged, and even, without remorse or trepidation, removed and replaced. The massive blood losses of which the liver was notoriously capable have been tamed, controlled, and allayed.

But progress has not been linear nor has it been parochial. Through fits of stops and starts and spread over centuries, understanding of the anatomic mélange that we have come to know as liver parenchyma in all its venous, arterial, and biliary intrigue slowly emerged as a rational partitioning of liver elements into (now) recognizable segments, sectors, and "lobes" (more properly, of course, "hemi-livers"). Contributions have literally been worldwide, from Europe, Asia, and the Americas through a myriad of investigator-surgeons, many of whom were simply inquisitive generalists who, once it could be done painlessly and aseptically, separated the tissues of the abdominal wall to delve into the recesses of the viscera, into territory formerly deadly and forbidden. It was here that a seemingly natural curiosity about that large reddish organ so apparently central to human metabolic workings expanded to boldly unravel the inner environment of this most mysterious of organs.

This work is not meant to be an exhaustive clinical review of current practices in liver surgery. Instead the authors have attempted to provide an admittedly rough sojourn through the pivotal moments and times that led to our present understanding of liver anatomy and surgery. The trail was roughly hewn with turns and twists, disappointments and successes that typifies scientific progress in medicine and surgery. We highlight those pioneers who, unintentionally, took courageous steps that furthered our ability as healers to offer hope to patients faced with conditions that had formerly defied treatment—cirrhosis, liver cancer, metastatic liver disease. In so telling, we used vignettes to illustrate and scientific literature to rationalize the numerous anecdotes that, together, comprised progress.

And of course liver surgery did not develop in a vacuum. It was the product of those monumental advances in medicine that suddenly provided abilities and opportunities only previously dreamed: general anesthesia, antisepsis, asepsis, and blood transfusions. The operating rooms of the twentieth century were radically different than those theaters of the nineteenth, as much as surgeons of the past century were far different from the brusque, arrogant, and, yes, theatrical ones who were their illustrious predecessors. In the twentieth century operating rooms took on the trappings of a laboratory instead of stage, the surgeons able to carefully and precisely define their objective rather than exhibit the callousness and speed necessary to overcome the shrieks and wails of their awake patients. And, following the holocaust of World War II, "modern" anesthesia came of age so that the operating rooms became well-orchestrated exhibitions of joint expertise and support. All fell under the watchful gaze of anesthetists who furnished the hemodynamic support for procedures and critical as liver resection and, then, liver transplantation. In so doing, surgeons were allowed to focus on the meticulous anatomic unweaving that now characterized the detailed labor necessary for eradication of deep-seated diseases. Those that focused on this organ and its mysteries developed a new particularization of general surgery, that subspecialty now representing yet another branch of the surgical tree. Through their efforts to define, analyze, minutely dissect, and innovate—based on the sound anatomic and physiologic endeavors of their forbearers (and, yes, their trials and errors)—manipulation of this organ, what the ancient Greeks considered the mysterious seat of the soul, has become a matter of distinctly corporal and common practice.

Jackson, MS   Thomas S. Helling
Villejuif, France   Daniel Azoulay

Contents

Chapter 1
Introduction

In injuries of the liver, as well as in resections of this organ, hemostasis presents the greatest difficulties

Professor Carl Garre, 1907

And ready-witted Prometheus [Zeus] bound with inextricable bonds, cruel chains, and drove a shaft through his middle, and set on him a long-winged eagle, which used to eat his immortal liver; but by night the liver grew as much again everyway as the long-winged bird devoured in the whole day

Hesiod's Theogony 521–526 [1]

In Greek mythology Prometheus, as punishment for defying Zeus and stealing fire to give to the human race, was chained to a rock in the Caucasus where, helpless to resist, an eagle pecked away by day at his liver only for it to regenerate at night and the ordeal repeated the next day. Such a torment extended not to the physical pain suffered, of which there seemed not a great amount, but to the spiritual, for the liver, for the Greeks, was considered the seat of the soul. So it was psychological torture, not physical, that plagued Prometheus, his very soul—his essence—violated but not destroyed, its capacity for renewal virtually immortal.

Yet, surgeons would not be so lucky as the long-winged eagle of Prometheus, both bird and man seemingly unaffected by the daily nibbling into blood-rich liver tissue. For surgeons—these gallant healers of antiquity—meddling in affairs of the liver was not meant as punishment but as salvation. And the elusive soul, if indeed the liver were its home, would be a formidable opponent, its invasion an unnerving task. In truth, the liver was a tarnished soul, host to an array of lethal diseases—tumors, cysts, and infections. The price to be paid from those intent to relieve suffering within, even by the most facile technicians, was usually exsanguination. Forays into the veritable seat of life–the heart—proved less deadly.

Within the liver coursed veins so large and thin-walled that violation produced a hemorrhage of such magnitude and virulence that death quickly followed. The operator stood helpless to comprehend a jungle of crisscrossing anatomy so unforgiving

T. S. Helling, D. Azoulay, *Historical Foundations of Liver Surgery*, https://doi.org/10.1007/978-3-030-47095-1_1

that sutures were of little avail, as dark blood poured from diminishing reservoirs. And the pale victim receded into the throes of profound shock until no pulse at all could be felt. Soon life fled; an experience so distasteful that most surgeons vowed never to return. Age old literature reported such adventures, hepatic wounds belching forth great volumes of venous blood, the task of hemostasis nigh impossible. Only by the most genteel of suturing could compression be achieved to staunch the flow, by then the lucky surgeon beaded with sweat near collapse himself, his patient pallid but blissfully unaware. Replacement of spent blood, of course, inconceivable; such miracles awaited courageous pioneers—patients and doctors—of the Twentieth Century. Without replenishment all peered down with subdued hopes to see if somehow their patient could rebound, mobilizing reserves that, for the time, escaped understanding. In 1897 noted surgeon and Boston Brahmin John Wheelock Elliot of the Massachusetts General Hospital, after completing an admittedly limited liver resection, noted in rather civil terms that "bleeding was profuse" (the patient apparently survived) [2].[1] Yet, reports of operative death rates over 60% were the norm, exsanguination the likely terminal event. In his chapter on liver surgery in Warren and Gould's *International Textbook of Surgery* Elliot would caution: "The organ is so friable, so full of gaping vessels, and so evidently incapable of being sutured, that it has always seemed impossible successfully to manage large wounds in its substance." As a result, in his mind, patient selection was imperative. "Only primary cancer as a single nodule is suitable for operation", he wrote [4]. It would be a full half century from the close of the *Belle Époque* before surgeons had at their means an understanding of the convoluted anatomy and an array of resources to compensate for the sanguine bloodlettings their surgery would produce.

To be sure, surgeons at the dawn of the Twentieth Century were a different breed of physician. With the advent of general anesthesia and use of aseptic techniques much more intricate operations were possible, delving into structures with the patience and painstaking efforts only dreamed about a half century before. There was now an air of caution in breaching those deeper, internal zones, a valid concern of whether such adventures would truly impact the course of disease. Even aside from the rampant infections of previous decades, surgeons were keenly aware of the consequences of their cutting. The one exception was cancer. Only surgery could effect a cure in those days before blood-borne cytotoxic agents. The wider the cut, the more likely the cure. And with refinements in anesthesia and supportive care, the cuts could be quite generous. Perhaps too generous, some felt. By mid-Century caution was advised. The fabled French surgeon René Leriche wrote:

> Ablation surgery is beautiful only sportively speaking: from the biological point of view, it is brutal, unnatural, and it is basically a poor therapy that cures the diseased organs by permanently removing them. We must have other ambitions for the future [5].

---

[1] Doctor Elliot indeed had a rich heritage. His great-grandfather had soldiered at Bunker Hill. A fastidious and orderly surgeon, he was of the mind that no operation should take more than 1 h, and often operated in his patient's homes. A master of the aseptic laparotomy, his surgical results were superb regardless of the site. See also Ernest Codman [3].

But little did Leriche know that not 20 years later the most dreaded of visceral organs, the liver, would be hacked, partitioned, and, yes, even completely removed in order to cure disease. It would be an odyssey of adventure filled with some of the most notable surgeons of the Twentieth Century, not barbarous types as Leriche may have thought, but true scientists and entrepreneurs who would advance the understanding of the liver and its central role in life itself. Perhaps those "other ambitions" for which Leriche had hoped would be far beyond his expectations.

References

1. Hesiod (1943) Theogony. In: Hesiod (ed) The Homeric hymns and Homerica with an english translation by Hugh G. Evelyn-White. Harvard University Press, Cambridge, MA, p 117
2. Elliot JW (1897) Surgical treatment of tumor of the liver with the report of a case. Ann Surg 26:83–95
3. Codman EA (1928) John Wheelock Elliot, M.D. N Engl J Med 198:994–1004
4. Warren JC, Pearce Gould A (1902) The international text-book of surgery. W.B. Saunders & Co, Philadelphia, pp 452–453
5. Leriche R (1945) La Chirurgie a l'Ordre de la Vie. La Presse francaise et etrangere, Paris, p 38

Chapter 2
The Bold Adventure of Lortat-Jacob

Jean-Louis Lortat-acob (1908–1992) cut an imposing figure, a man of amazing physical strength and endurance. Outwardly aloof and reserved, this demeanor actually concealed a character of great modesty [1]. To intimates he was warm, friendly, and prone to loving anecdotes. He was a man humbled by his accomplishments; loathe to inwardly acknowledge what was so obvious to others. Outwardly he was a task master, intent on quiet perfection, disciplined by his upbringing. Jean-Louis was born into a medical family in 1908, the fourth of six children whose father was a dermatologist in Paris. From a strong Catholic family (he was educated by the Dominicans), Jean-Louis began the study of medicine and was drawn to surgery. He trained under the grand masters of surgery, Louis Bazy, Pierre Brocq, and Henri Mondor, among others [2], facilitated, possibly, by his father's professional and personal acquaintances with these men. The young Lortat-Jacob joined the faculty of the *Hôpital St-Louis* in 1944 as a prosector and assistant to Professor Bazy. Despite his sorties into hepatic surgery, the name Lortat-Jacob is inextricably linked to surgery of the esophagus. Jean-Louis performed the first esophagectomy in France in 1944 via a thoracic approach [3]. He left *the Hôpital St-Louis* for the *Hôpital Broussais* where he joined the prestigious surgical team of Professor François de Gaudart d'Allaines (1892–1974). Gaudart d'Allaines had been a pioneer in foregut surgery, including a fascination with the liver and biliary system. This may have stimulated Lortat-Jacob's interest. It was at this time that he may first have pondered the daunting approach to surgery of the liver, and thus acquainted himself with the anatomy of the Glissonean pedicles and hepatic veins, learning temperance and patience at the side of his mentor.

The *Hôpital Broussais* itself was a remarkable edifice. It had been built in less than 3 months in 1883, erected in the 14th arrondissement on the southern outskirts of Paris, straddling the communes more colloquially known as Gentilly and Montrouge, those formerly rural habitats of monasteries and goldsmiths and sites of royal hunts. An ideal location, it was said, for the terrible cholera epidemic that swept through Paris that very year: "the most perfect arrangements, from a sanitary

© The Editor(s) (if applicable) and The Author(s), under exclusive license to
Springer Nature Switzerland AG 2020
T. S. Helling, D. Azoulay, *Historical Foundations of Liver Surgery*,
https://doi.org/10.1007/978-3-030-47095-1_2

point of view" [4]. Initially designated as a hospital for seafarers, the name was changed to "Broussais" in 1885, in honor of the renowned François Joseph Victor Broussais (1772–1838), physician and surgeon of the Empire. Piece by piece from 1928 until 1940 the hospital was rebuilt. In 1935 the new facility opened under the surgical leadership of the *debonair* Gaudart d'Allaines, "a man of gentle manners … who emanated great charm" [5]. It was there that Gaudart d'Allaines began his innovating work in foregut surgery and operations on the biliary system. Later, after time in the United States with Alfred Blalock, Gaudart d'Allaines shifted his interest to operations on the heart. But even more significant was his insistence that clinical surgery be accompanied by parallel efforts in research, perfecting operative techniques in animal models before embarking on human trials, soon to characterize French surgical practice.

On a Tuesday morning, October 16, 1951 Professor Lortat-Jacob entered the operating room of the *Hôpital Broussais* and opened the abdomen of a 42 year old pianist whom his assistant Henry Robert had examined and found a palpable tumor in the right hypochondrium. Their suspicions were that this represented a hydatid cyst of the liver; their intent complete extirpation. Instead, upon entering the abdominal cavity, the surgeons found three tumors involving the right lobe of the liver, two of which were larger than grapefruits and the third the size of an orange. As far as Lortat-Jacob was aware, no one had attempted total removal of the right lobe of the liver, which, at the time, was defined topographically as the mass of liver to the right of the falciform ligament. The fear was that of exsanguinating hemorrhage or, perhaps, liver failure by leaving a too small amount of liver tissue behind. To date no European seemed to have a firm grasp on precisely how to split the liver in half without voluminous hemorrhage. It seemed reasonable to think, though, that some control of blood flow into the liver at the hilum and control of blood leaving the liver at the confluence of hepatic veins just above the liver might afford a more or less "regulated" attempt.

And on that day in October, 1951 Lortat-Jacob had exactly that in mind. His assault was rehearsed; his knowledge of the liver detailed. He was the consummate abdominal surgeon. Just as he had perfected in his surgery of gastric tumors, using a radical left *abdomino-thoracique* incision, Lortat-Jacob propped up his patient's right flank and sliced into the right chest, across the costal margin, and into the abdomen, dividing the diaphragm and laying bare the entire right lobe of the liver.[1] It was only then that the true nature of his patient's condition was unveiled: three tumors in the right lobe. It would take an entire right lobectomy to remove them all. For such a momentous operation Lortat-Jacob would entrust anesthesia only to his seasoned colleague and friend, the anesthetist Brunet d'Aubiac. Only then did he begin. And here would be what set Lortat-Jacob apart. Before invading liver substance, he would control blood flow. Contrary to the popular approach of liver surgeons before him who too often plunged into liver parenchyma and suffered the

---

[1] Lortat-Jacob's presented this case before the Société Nationale Française de Gastro-Entérologie which published the proceedings as "Hepatectomie Lobaire Droite Réglée Pour Tumeur Maligne Secondaire" [6]. The French medical journal *Presse Medicale* would soon publish the case in their April 16, 1952 issue [7].

wrath of torrential hemorrhage, Lortat-Jacob intended to stifle this tendency by interrupting blood borne pathways first. After securing hilar control of the vessels and ducts, Lortat-Jacob mobilized the bulbous right liver by dividing the peritoneal attachments, gaining access to the retrohepatic inferior vena cava. He then divided the minor hepatic veins to the inferior vena cava and then carefully encircled and divided the right hepatic vein. This completely freed the right lobe for removal. The parenchyma just to the right of the falciform ligament was transected—largely by finger-fracture—ligating intra-parenchymal branches in the process. Working steadily towards the inferior vena cave he and his assistant Robert included the *lobe carré* (quadrate lobe, Couinaud's segment IVa) and divided its delicate vascular attachments to the hilum. Lortat-Jacob then lifted the massive right lobe from the patient, having performed what, in later terminology, would be a trisectionectomy (five of Couinaud's eight segments). The left lobe, Couinaud segments I, II, and III, was no bigger than a fist (*"n'est pas plus gros que le poing"*). In his words, despite widespread fears, *"Il n'y a aucune hemorrhagie"*—there was no bleeding [7]. With regard to liver function, notwithstanding the alarmingly small liver remnant, there were few perturbations, and the patient was alive and well 3 months later. The tumors proved to be metastases from either a biliary or a pancreatic carcinoma.

Bravo! The feat was acclaimed as a major advance in visceral surgery. "I would like to stress the high level of interest of this exceptional communication by my friend Lortat-Jacob. As far as I know, this is an original observation, not only in France, but also in all the medical literature", so exclaimed his mentor, Professor d'Allaines, commenting on Lortat-Jacob's presentation before the *Société Nationale Française de Gastro-Entérologie* which met on March 31, 1952 [6]. Fifty years later the feat was still celebrated. Jacques Belghiti declared in 2003 (perhaps a bit effusively) that "[t]he first anatomical right resection" by Lortat-Jacob forecast the eventual application of his technique to transplantation and, specifically, split-liver transplantation: "Lortat-Jacob conceived the evolution of liver surgery announcing one of the most important advancements in liver transplantation over 50 years ago [split-liver transplantation to ease the donor shortage]" [8].

Indeed, it was a widely publicized affair, and for good reason. Lortat-Jacob had ushered in new dimensions of visceral surgery, an era that had begun almost 100 years prior. The abdomen had been successfully broached since the time of Christian Albert Theodor BIllroth (1829–1894) and his famous *Chirurgischen Klinik* (Surgical Clinic) at the *Allgemeine Krankenhaus* (General Hospital) in Vienna. All was possible now that the patients were blissfully anesthetized by the new inhalation agent ether and its cousin, chloroform. And Lister's observations on antisepsis could even prevent disastrous postoperative infections. As a result, by the close of the nineteenth century esophagus and stomach and colon were well within the grasp of still frock-coated, cigar-smoking surgeons. Yet one organ paled the enthusiasts of the *fin de siècle*. Uncontrolled hemorrhage was still the unwelcome outcome of explorations into the depths of the liver, hemorrhage so persistent that death was a familiar visitor, much to the vexation of the emboldened surgeon. This organ and its seeming morass of aimless and flimsy blood vessels defied control, and gave pause to even the most ambitious operator.

Oh yes there had been adventurers, despite the trepidations. There had been pioneers, some who failed and some who succeeded—all contributing to that mosaic of scientific progress. Many remained in the shadows of obscurity even after their lone achievements and momentary brilliance. But all would unknowingly pave the way for the pivotal entrance of Lortat-Jacob and modern liver surgery.

References

1. Ribet M (1992) Necrologie: Jean-Louis Lortat-Jacob (1908-1992). Chirurgie 118:583–584
2. Boutelier P (1996) Eloge de Jean-Louis Lortat-Jacob. Chirurgie 121:589–596
3. Launois B (1990) Symposium dedicated to professor Jean-Louis Lortat-Jacob: introduction. Dig Surg 7:77–78
4. Tomkins H (1885) Some brief notes on the late outbreak of cholera in Paris. Lancet 1:511–512
5. Debré R (1974) François de Gaudart d'Allaines. La Nouvelle Revue Des Deux Mondes:568–572
6. Lortat-Jacob J-LR (1952) Hepatectomie Lobaire Droite Reglee Pour Tumeur Maligne Secondaire. Arch Mal App Digestif 41:662–667
7. Lortat-Jacob J-L, Robert H-G (1952) Hepatectomie Droite Reglee. Presse Med 60:549–551
8. Belghiti J (2003) The first anatomical right resection announcing liver donation. J Hepatology 39:475–479

Chapter 3
The Liver: Impossible Salvations

Outside Hamburg Germany on a summer day in 1835 a 10 year old boy was playing in the garden with an open knife in his right pants pocket. As young boys will do, he was in a hurry, stooped, perhaps to tie a shoe, and lost his balance, falling to his knees and then, awkwardly, flat on his stomach. The knife did not flatten with the fall but penetrated his abdomen, obliquely from his naval into the right upper quadrant. He saw the blood, panicked, and ran home. When first examined he had a sizeable bleeding wound on the right side, with a strange, bloody piece of tissue hanging out of the opening. The knife was intact and was removed. Taken to a local surgeon, the boy was wrapped in a compressive bandage but advised to go to the *Allgemeinen Krankenhaus*—the large general hospital—in Hamburg. There he was examined by Doctor Fricke and his team. Fricke described a peculiar reddish structure that lay poking through the wound on a stalk-shaped attachment covered with a bloody coagulum. It was clear to all that this was a piece of the boy's liver that had been divided by the knife blade. The hanging piece of liver was carefully excised and the stalk was treated with "anti-inflammatory" ointments and salves. The fortunate lad recovered quickly and was restored to full health within a few weeks. Years later, with the death of the, now, adult man, an autopsy in fact did reveal that the sliced piece of tissue had indeed been a portion of the liver [1].

Indeed, most early encounters with the liver were in the form of trauma, and then only to staunch the rather alarming bleeding that so often occurred or, as happened to Professeur Fricke's young patient, to complete a near amputation of a dangling part. From the dawn of written history the organ of Prometheus has been connected to bounteous and frightful bleeding, particularly when wounded. Homer, in his saga of the siege of Troy, noted three separate occasions when the liver was skewered during close combat. That famed warrior Achilles, wreaking havoc among the Trojan ranks singled out Alastor's son Tros, who, sensing his fate, collapsed to clasp Achilles knees. Achilles, unmoved, thrust his sword into Tros' midsection, slicing into his liver that, partially severed, slid from the wound and spilled dark blood drenching his body and "darkness enfolded him and his spirit left him". And the

Greek hero Odysseus, on his 10-year sojourn from Troy to Ithaca, cornered in the Cyclops' cave, contemplated thrusting his sharp sword below the Cyclops' breast ὅθι φρένες φπαρ ἔχουσι—where the midriff (diaphragm) holds the liver. "A wound in that place", the ancients considered, "would not permit life to continue even for a moment" [2, 3].

The First Century Roman physician (or encyclopedist) Cornelius Celsus (25 BC—50 CE), in his extensive compendium *De Medicina* wrote about penetrating abdominal wounds and advised physicians on the treatment of eviscerating injuries. However he noted that wounds of the liver resulted in "great effusion of blood under the right side of the hypochondra … also, bilious vomiting is added" "It is impossible to save a patient when the base of the brain, or the heart, or the gullet, or the porta of the liver … is wounded", he stressed [4].

Armenius Marcellinus, a soldier in the army of Byzantine emperor Julian the Apostate (331–336 CE), recalled how his commander fell battling the Persians in 336. Caught in a swarm of "fugitives" and without body armor due to the heat, the 31 year old Julian was struck by a cavalryman's spear just under the hypocondrium. Marcellinus said the spear penetrated and was "trapped in the depths of his liver". Julian, slipping from his horse, was weakened and "troubled by the great issue of blood". Taken to his tent the young warrior-king bravely conversed with his aides and camp philosophers as if in full command of his senses, but suddenly the terrible wound opened up and blood poured forth. Julian, no doubt taken into shock, could no longer maintain his composure and quietly passed away [5].

These scenarios were likely commonplace occurrences in the medieval world. Only infrequently, with fortuitous evisceration of part of the liver, could surgeons address the troublesome bleeding and staunch hemorrhage with ligature or compression. In most cases, these injuries proved fatal. Survivable trauma was restricted to wounds of the anterior liver—those lacerations of relatively slender liver substance that bled only from peripheral branches of portal vein or hepatic veins. Deeper injuries that opened up larger vessels were much more ominous. "The parts which give many indications of death when a wound occurs in them are: the bladder, the brain, the heart, the kidneys, the liver, the diaphragm, the stomach, and the small intestine", so wrote the Italian surgeon, friar and Bishop of Cervia, Theodoric Borgognoni (1205–1298) in the thirteenth Century.

Heavily influenced by the writings of Theodoric and the Eleventh Century Islamic scholar Avicenna, the French surgeon Henri de Mondeville (c. 1260–1320) compiled a vast resource for contemporary surgical thought and practice in a lengthy tome entitled *Cyrugia* (later, *La Chirurgie* in its French translation). The liver was felt central to the digestive process, a principal organ filled with blood supplied by a maze of veins originating from the intestine. Centuries before, the blood-engorged liver was thought by Galen of Pergamon to be the seat of sanguification—it was here that the rich red blood was made. It would be this literal blood reservoir that, when injured, would pour forth voluminous amounts of crimson liquid, the type de Mondville reported issues "with violence … as the water brought by a lead-pipe flows from a fountain". In arresting such hemorrhage, the situation was often so desperate that, in those heavily spirited times—surgeon and priest must collaborate: who to proceed first, the surgeon and his attempts to stop such hemorrhage or the priest to hear confession from a subject likely soon to die. Which to attend first: body or soul? In other respects, de Mondeville's discussion of wounds was extensive, from proper bandaging to suturing to stemming of blood flow. For chest and abdominal penetrating thrusts de Mondeville recommended that any foreign bodies be removed and that the wounds be closed fast to prevent ingress of putrefied air. But there were some wounds, in his experience and those of others, that were not salvageable. These were hopeless injuries where any treatment would be futile. So he wrote:

> These wounds are necessarily fatal: wounds that surround the heart, wounds of the diaphragm, of the stomach, and of the liver. The reason that the wounds of the liver and spleen are lethal is that these organs perform a function necessary to the whole body and that they cannot exercise it when they are wounded, so the whole body perishes [6].

Hemorrhage almost certainly played a major role but, one would assume, the extent was often hidden by lack of external bleeding.

"The liver is principally made of blood", so copied the Italian Lanfranc of Milan (c. 1250–1306) in the fourteenth Century. And liberation of this blood had dire consequences. He admonished that "if the liver be hurt in the deep substance, then the liver shall lose all her workings and all the blood thereof that is the matter of the spirit disturbed and, by this manner, the spirit of life will be disturbed" (in essence, a fatal wound). Only those injuries to the liver that are "but little" and are fresh can be healed, he maintained [7].

The great Renaissance surgeon and anatomist Fabricius Hildanus (1560–1634) was considered the "Father of German Surgery". His attention to details of anatomy and operative technique put him on a par with Ambroise Paré. Those with less motivation, he contended, were idle misfits. "While the young surgeons should apply themselves to the study of Anatomy, they make music, read the owl-glass, drink, fornicate, enjoy themselves or adorn their rooms and waste their time", he wrote [8]. As for his own diligence, his chronicles of case histories are legendary. In *Observationum et Curationum Chirurgicarum Centuriae* Hildanus speaks of a young Swiss nobleman struck in the "liver area" by a sword. "A piece of liver appeared at the entrance of the wound, which was fished out unhindered". The gentleman fully recovered, but some years later was consumed with fever. Fabricius visited him and found him "suffering greatly" and lamenting that now he should be plagued with fever when only a few years before a surgeon had miraculously pulled out and severed a piece of his liver. When the poor soul died, Fabricius opened his abdomen and found that some of the "lower lobe" of the liver had indeed been cut off but had healed, covered by a scar—perhaps an unrecognized result of regenerative capacity [9].[1]

But through the ages, trauma still commanded attention of surgeons, particularly in the recesses of the abdomen where deadly injuries and skyrocketing lethality beckoned surgeon emboldened by antisepsis and anesthesia. Hemorrhage during liver trauma and liver surgery loomed large among surgeons undertaking the task of hemostasis—the checking of blood loss. Uncontrollable bleeding was (and is) every

---

[1] Parenthetically, Schaefer, a noted German medical historian, and his wife were both killed in the devastating bombing of Darmstadt, Germany, the night of September 11/12. 1944. His vast archives were destroyed as well.

surgeon's nightmare, especially that dark, welling blood coming from recesses in the cut surface of liver that seems to overflow the operative field. Soon evidence of dwindling life appears, a rapid, undulating, soft pulse replaces the robust bounding rhythm of minutes before. The patient takes on the look of distress. Surgeon Charles Bell wrote in 1816 "When the bleeding is extreme, and passing to a dangerous state, the paleness of the face is accompanied by an anxious wildness or delirious look, which should command immediate attention …" There is an unhappy, hasty search for open vessels, but unlike the brisk, easily identifiable hemorrhage from arteries, dozens of minute veins in the liver leak their purple contents forming one swirling bloody pool. The immediate recourse is compression—*le tamponnement* the French so wisely advised. Bell went on to say:

"When the bleeding … comes from deep parts—where it is dangerous to lay the bottom open—where not one large artery, but many lesser ones are wounded, then the sponge and graduated compress ought to be used …" [10]

Sometimes it was not enough. Before the era of blood replacement, failure to control bleeding allowed life to slip away as if humanity itself had drowned in the blood swamp the surgeon had created. Before long, pulse fades, heart beats slow until nothing but stillness descends and death in its pungent odor overcomes. It is then that surgeon steps back, speechless, and fears that he himself has robbed his subject of vigor, of existence; that he–and no one else–is transformed from Angel of Rescue to Angel of Death. He has become traitor to his profession. It is the antithesis of all he has aspired and for which he has trained.

While some claimed any attempt to operate for penetrating abdominal injuries was almost foolhardy, others felt differently. In America Dr. J. C. Massie of Houston, Texas operated on a seven-year old boy accidently shot in the right upper abdomen 4 days before. By enlarging the gunshot wound itself Dr. Massie was able excise almost "one half of the right lobe [of the liver], equal to twice the amount of the left". It had become "gangrenous" with a thick "grumous" appearance and threatened the boy's life. "I felt great apprehension in excising the amount I was necessarily compelled to do", he stressed, quoting a noted military surgeon as saying "A deep wound of the liver is as fatal as if the heart itself was engaged." The boy apparently made a complete recovery [11]. In another instance, a rather intrepid Henry C. Dalton, professor of surgery at Marion Sims College of Medicine (now Saint Louis University School of Medicine) in 1888 reported success in operating on a patient suffering a laceration of the liver, which he deftly closed with sutures placed "a good distance from the edge of the wound, … and, of carrying them *deeply* into the substance of the liver". He then reviewed 69 cases of laparotomy for gunshot wounds—a process he referred to as "abdominal section for traumatism" and recorded survivable success in five of 10 liver wounds (with an overall mortality from all abdominal wounds of 59%). Thomas Morton, of Philadelphia extended this series to 234 patients by 1890 including 24 with liver injuries (13 deaths, 54%). Again, catgut suture and simple packing were procedures advocated [12, 13].[2]

---

[2] In Morton's report American surgeons experienced a 65% mortality for all injuries while "foreign surgeons" (largely European) faced a 48% mortality.

Yes, the liver was a formidable organ, indeed. The punctures and splits endured by human violence were often unforgiving, despite heroic efforts of audacious surgeons spoiling for a fight to save dwindling lives. Its substance forbad common use of sutures, bleeding welled from its depths, and compression merely tried the perserverance of surgeons anxious to somehow stem its incessant hemorrhage. There was little excitement among even the most talented of operators to test their mettle against this bloody structure.

References

1. Fricke JC (1836) Bericht über die in die chirurgische Abteilung des allgemeinen Krankenhauses aufgenommenen Kranken, vom Juli bis September 1835. Zeitschrift fur die gesammte Medicin:315–316
2. Homer (1995) Odyssey. Harvard University Press, Cambridge, p 301, Book 9
3. Galen (1968) On the usefulness of the parts of the body. Cornell University Press, Ithaca, p 231
4. Celsus (1938) De Medicina. Harvard University Press, Cambridge, p 26, Book V
5. Rolfe JC (1940) Ammianus Marcellinus: Rerum Gestarum. Harvard University Press, Cambridge, pp 6–23, XXV. 3
6. Nicaise E (1893) Chirurgie de Maitre Henri de Mondeville. Felix Alcan, Paris, p 247, 370–372
7. Lanfranc (1894) Science of Cirurgie (translated by Robert v. Fleischhacker). Kegan Paul, Trench, Trubner & Co, London, p 172
8. Jones EW (1960) The life and works of Guihelmus Fabricius Hildanus (1560-1634). Med Hist 4:196–209
9. Schaefer RJ (1914) Wilhelm Fabry's von Hilden (Fabricus Hildanus). Johann Ambrosius Barth, Leipzig, pp 48–51
10. Bell C (1816) A system of operative surgery, Volume 2. George Goodwin and Sons, Hartford, p 391
11. Massie JC (1852) Wounds of the liver—excision of a large portion of the right lobe. New Orleans Med Surg J 9:146–148
12. Dalton HC (1888) Gunshot wound of stomach and liver treated by laparotomy and suture of visceral wounds with recovery. Ann Surg 8:81–100
13. Morton TS (1890) Abdominal section for traumatism with tables of two hundred and thirty-five cases. JAMA 14:1–16

Chapter 4
The Art of Operating

Yet elective procedures on the liver awaited developments in surgery that enhanced comfort of the patient and outcome of the operation. These happenings had a profound influence on surgeons and their willingness to stretch the limits of daring especially in an organ as unforgiving as the liver. Indeed, the Nineteenth Century saw an explosion of interest in the surgical arts. From an era of near-butchery when operations were done as rapidly as possible on patients held down by assistants for fear the luckless subject would panic and bolt, the use of general ether anesthesia revolutionized ability of surgeons to dive deeper into the human substance and open up heretofore forbidding regions of disease and disorder.

While in the first half of the Nineteenth Century, Paris was the darling of the American set who traveled to Europe to learn at hands of the great masters, Berlin and Vienna soon drew those fickle tourists after mid-century. Attitudes for instruction in Paris had changed since the February Revolution of 1848. Private one-on-one instructions by eager *internes* was no longer allowed, citing risks to the patient. What had formerly been a magnet for foreign students was now impossible, and the lowly American but one of many who must follow the crowds of physicians rounding on hospitalized patients. By law Germany had usurped Parisian enticements for medical tourism. Private instructions were now sanctioned by the state and access to a wealth of patients and pathology in Berlin and Vienna virtually unlimited. Bostonian David Lincoln described his experiences in the Austrian capital in 1871: "The foreign physician sees and profits from the young and ambitious talent that abounds here; he comes in contact, four or five hours a day, with various teachers, each anxious to secure to him the full benefit of his trouble and time, each fully competent to instruct and furnished with abundant examples" [1]. German, Swiss, and Austrian surgeons were intent on bringing surgery into the laboratory, even to the point of considering human subjects "material" and objects of science. Despite the denigration of patients observed by American visitors, most visiting physicians eagerly attended lectures and demonstrations that, at times, dehumanized their focus of instruction. It was here that the pathology of Virchow, the cunning of

Theodor Billroth, and the precision of Emil Theodor Kocher (1841–1907) were on display—a true melding of laboratory science and clinical acumen. Surgery was, in these hands, a masterpiece of art, no longer slashing and daring, but meticulous, plodding, as if slow strokes of paint on fine brushes were being applied to canvas.

It was indeed a time of industrious unification for the German federation. Timothy Lenoir reported: "The best interest of the state was an economic policy supporting material well-being of its citizens. This was accomplished through construction of the Zollverein, encouragement of industry, and free trade within the economic boundaries of the German states". No less medicine, which captured the attention of the rigorous and logical German mind. "Medicine was in a building period in which it was attempting to understand better the facts of medical experience with new methods and apparatus adapted from other empirical sciences, particularly physics, chemistry, and physiology" [2].

These men were part of a new generation of surgery, surgeons in the era of antisepsis, asepsis, and anesthesia, where speed and aplomb were qualities no longer needed. Now all was aimed at sterility, fine, deliberate motions, and an intent to cure, to radicalize—in the sense of completeness—operations so as to totally eradicate disease and afford a chance of full recovery. In his address before the British Medical Association in August, 1900 Frederick Treves described the surgeon of the Nineteenth Century as a man steeped in learning, a master of his handiwork, his skills having undergone a metamorphosis reaching the level of the unexpected. And anesthesia, he emphasized, had "greatly extended the domain of surgery by rendering possible operations which before could have been only dreamt about" [3].[1]

Such men as the illustrious Ernst von Bergmann (1836–1907) stepped forward, one who no longer subscribed to the old idiom that "the operation has been achieved. God will heal you!" The act of surgery was not, as he had experienced in his training, "a bloody act" with little regard to the wound, only to rapid hemostasis. Von Bergmann would now advocate meticulous attention to asepsis. "What good does it help the patient that he has been artfully and excellently operated, if the admirable operation does not allow him recovery?" Surgeons must accept responsibility for the operation and the total healing of the patient. Science and technology will guide a surgeon's actions, not just bravado and speed [4]. It would be the mark of German ascendancy in the surgical arts. Traveling American surgeon Nicholas Senn would marvel at the great Theodor Kocher in Bern, Switzerland, his meticulous, diligent technique a signature quality.

> I consider him in every sense of the word the greatest surgeon I have ever seen. He is an accomplished scholar, an accurate careful diagnostician, a bold and dexterous operator and a born teacher … He is of slender build, and his whole appearance suggests thoughtfulness and hard work [Kocher was only 47 years old at the time] [5].

---

[1]A remarkable summation of the transformation of surgery and surgeons engendered by asepsis and anesthesia.

Indeed Germanic countries were flourishing. The celebrated Theodor Billroth (1829–1894) had proclaimed Berlin the new Paris:

> Finally, in view of my earlier remarks concerning German surgery, I will add that it is now at a level which is completely equal to that of the rest of the world, if not more important than France at present. We are now setting out to train scientifically in surgery, not to travel to Paris [6].

Perhaps, as historian Thomas Schlich contends, it was the introduction of asepsis as a necessary requisite for safe surgery—to combat the deadly effects of wound bacteria that prompted a realignment of surgery and laboratory science, soon to typify Germanic medicine. Schlich concluded that "by the early twentieth century laboratory science had become more central to surgery than ever before … It enabled a new time regime, allowing for more thorough and technically demanding operations" [7].

Surgery would not only be the "hand work" of ancient times.[2] Despite Billroth's 1863 claim that "Only one thing is required of the surgeon … namely, the art of operating" [6],[3] surgery would become a science integrating with other studies of anatomy, pathology, and physiology. A revolution was in the making, in large part due to the unraveling of the mysteries of miasmas and wound sepsis. It was not air itself that promoted evils of suppuration, but the particles harbored within and carried aloft that settle in open cuts and slashes and wrought their damage forthwith. Joseph Lister's claim of airborne pathogens as causative agents and use of the antiseptic carbolic acid radically altered outcomes of surgical procedures. However, not only was Lister a strong advocate of his antiseptic regimen, he also stressed attention to all details of operation, diametrically opposed to contemporary surgeons who not only questioned the validity of his microbial theories but also failed to appreciate minute ramifications of their sometimes brutish approach to tissue handling. Lister was the ultimate model of professionalism. As Michael Worboys emphasized in his treatise, "Lister's professionalism was seen not only in his demeanor and character, but also in his operative performance at every level; no detail was too insignificant for his attention" [8]. It became the moral obligation of surgeons to ensure optimal care for their patients. Now, surgeons and the laboratory became inexorably linked. On his arrival in Berlin, Bergmann developed a fast friendship with Kocher. Kocher's pivotal work in the laboratory on identification and eradication of microbes extended far beyond Lister's empirical recommendations. Verification of sterility was not a clinical measure but could only be obtained under rigid, controlled conditions in the laboratory and had a critical role in unimpeded wound healing. Bergmann was of the mind that there were several elements of surgery that must be commanded—antisepsis, hemostasis, wound closure, and drainage. All to be verified through close cooperation with laboratory scientists.

---

[2] The word "surgery" (Latin *chirurgia*) is thought to arise from the ancient Greek χείρ (hand) + έργον (work) = "handwork"

[3] Billroth, *Die allgemeine chirurgische*, 3

The surgery of the present is by no means art or craft alone. Neither artful talent nor the conscientious and embarrassing observance of the instructions of a beloved Master make them powerful. It became what it is and attained the position which it occupies at the moment among the sister disciplines, merely through the scientific method ... [9]

Experimentalism had become the rage. In physiology French scientists and surgeons Francois Magendie and Claude Bernard performed carefully crafted investigations in physiology in their Paris laboratories, insisting that only there could sufficiently controlled work uncover the true machinery of man (For further reading into the maturation of experimental physiology see [10]). With the daunting task of surgery on such an intimidating organ as the liver, the laboratory seemed a reasonable place to perfect techniques and bring to light consequences of assault on this ill-tempered organ.

It was under this philosophy that the Romanian Themistocles Gluck (1853–1942) began his animal work in liver surgery. As a young man, Gluck had learned experimental science under the tutelage of the great Rudolf Virchow and Bernhard von Langenbeck. His clinical experiences had taught him that "it would be hard to dare a surgeon to undertake liver surgery in humans." Animal work must first be done, he insisted. While studying with Virchow, he devised a series of experiments on liver surgery in the rabbit, cat, and dog in which by manipulating the portal flow, he was able to successfully remove one-third of the liver without apparent harm to the animals and two-thirds of livers with survival for several days. Occlusion of the portal vein, heretofore a lethal maneuver, and infusion of saline solution via the jugular vein to restore circulating volume proved instrumental in the animals" survival. "I think it probable", he wrote of his work, "that, after these experiments, practical surgery on the liver can expect to benefit" [11].

Yet other Germans were piecemeal teasing the liver, attacking and stripping away its appendages in ever more brazen maneuvers. Carl Johann August Langenbuch (1846–1901) was appointed Director of Surgery at the *Lazarus Kranckenhaus* (Hospital) in Berlin at the young age of 27. It was at the *Lazarus*, in 1882, that Langenbuch performed the first cholecystectomy in humans on a 43 year old man suffering for years from biliary colic. Heretofore, gallbladder troubles were usually dealt with by cholecystotomy, sometimes referred to as "cholecystostomy", first attempted around mid-century. Theodore Kocher had recommended this operation—suturing the opened gallbladder to the abdominal wall over cholecystotomy since he had observed a number of deaths with simple stone extraction and closure of the gallbladder [12]. A palpable, tender gallbladder felt below the ribcage was a prerequisite, and a short incision and opening of the gallbladder (with or without extraction of stones and suturing to the abdominal wall) would hopefully resolve an acute, debilitating condition.

As was so often the case in those days of explorations, new operations were only attempted on the drastically ill, those whose quality or quantity of life ebbed to the point of imminent deep depression or death. And this patient, referred by a colleague, Langenbuch knew was in desperate straits. Repeated painful attacks of colic over the years had crippled him, morphine barely provided relief. On occasion the poor man would simply faint from the agony. "[W]*ar er gemütlich sehr deprimirt ... und sähe einer düsteren Zukunft entgegen*" (he was likely very depressed … and looked forward to a gloomy future). Even more so, his condition was rapidly deteriorating. Weakness, weight loss (20 kg), and dependence on morphine all made for a risky undertaking. Langenbuch had witnessed a similar picture in a 40 year-old hospital administrator whose gallbladder attacks finally terminated in sepsis and death. Humble, attentive, and outwardly unassertive, he was held in great respect by his colleagues. Cholecystectomy, he knew, had been shunned by the surgical community because of a fear of unwanted complications and death. Yet, physiologically, there were situations where inflammation of the gallbladder was irreconcilable with recovery, where mere opening and stone removal might not eradicate the septic focus. He had practiced his operation on cadavers, exposing critical structures of the cystic duct and artery, ligation, and gentle removal of the structure from the underside of this liver. The operation took place on July 15, 1882. His approach was calculating, careful, with undue attention to asepsis because of the "novelty" of the case. All went well, just as in his cadaver dissections. The patient had a perfect recovery, pain subsided, appetite returned, and morphine eliminated [13].

And then, several years later, in 1887, Langenbuch encountered a young woman, 30 years old, hospitalized for erysipelas, who refused to be discharged because of a painful abdominal mass that she had endured for 8 years. She insisted: "*da ihr Leben doch keinen Werth für sie haben würde, wenn wir nicht ihren Bauch*"—"since life would not be worth living if he did not take care of the painful mass". Langenbuch could easily palpate the mass on examination and on January 13, 1887 opened her abdomen to find, what he called, hepatoptosis of the left side of her liver. This downward displacement of the liver had resulted in formation of a palpable tumor separated from the rest of the liver by a fibrous constricting band of tissue, and was the likely source of the woman's pain, engorged as it was, presumably from the constriction caused by her tight corset, a common practice in those days among fashionable girls.[4] It may have been that Langenbuch had read the experimental work of Gluck and felt confident of his ability to carry out such surgery in human subjects. He proceeded to remove the mass, apparently attached to the remaining liver by a bridge of fibrous tissue. The entire specimen weighed 370 g or about one-quarter of the liver. His description of the operation does not indicate any particular attempt to do an anatomic resection, nor does he describe any major vascular or biliary structures. On inspecting the cut surface, Langenbuch felt all vessels had been ligated and so chose to close the abdominal incision rather than exteriorizing the liver as some had advocated. However, the patient showed signs of internal bleeding that evening (she looked quite pale and apoplectic) and required an urgent re-operation. Indeed there was blood—the abdomen was full of it—and one weakly bleeding vessel. He evacuated the blood, ligated the bleeder, and again closed the abdomen. No further bleeding occurred, but she developed troublesome ascites needing two paracenteses. His patient finally left the hospital in February.

---

[4] It appears at the *fin de siècle* it was highly desirable for ladies to have a dramatic hour-glass figure; the smaller the waist the better. Corsets were commonly used to achieve this appearance and were tightened like laces of a shoe (*schnur -*) to constrict the abdomen just below the rib cage.

Fig. 4.1 Carl Langenbuch
(1846–1901).
Public domain

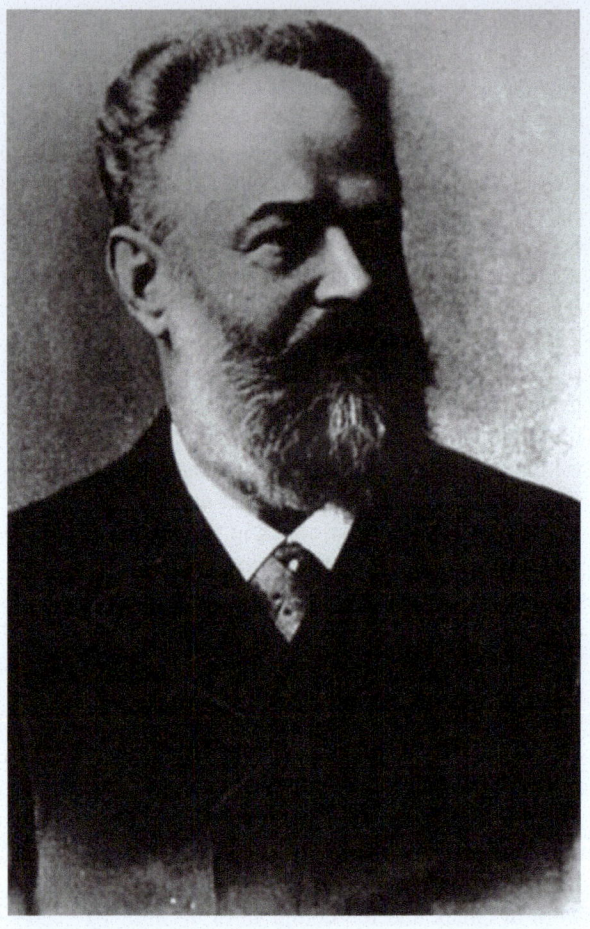

Langenbuch indeed ascribed the wearing of her tight corset as a possible cause of constricting her hepatoptic liver and creating the engorged liver mass. His labeling of this phenomenon—*schnurlappens*—loosely translated as a "bound" liver lobe, must have piqued the interest of the medical community [14].

Langenbuch was no stranger to liver surgery (Fig. 4.1). For surgeons of the late nineteenth Century primary concerns about liver pathology were not neoplasms or the peculiar conditions of his corseted patient in 1887, but the infectious dangers of bacterial liver abscesses and parasitic Echinococcal disease. In fact, he would publish his textbook on liver surgery in 1894 *Chirurgie der Leber und Gallenblase*. He would preface his discussion of the topic with an introductory statement, perhaps the vanguard declaration of a new and venturesome specialty:

> The gradual development of independent liver and gallbladder surgery, which has steadily begun in the last decades, and has become increasingly rapid, has prompted the surgeon to come to terms with the anatomy, physiology, and pathology. It is therefore not unreasonable

for more extensive versions of its surgery to preface it with an introduction commensurate
with this requirement, especially for the liver [15]⁵

Topographically, Langenbuch's depiction of external anatomy was entirely accurate. He maintained that the liver was composed of a large right (up to the falciform
ligament) and smaller left *Leberlappen*—liver lobes. Internally, he followed the
vascular depictions of the Austrian anatomist Hugo Rex, the main portal vein
branching to the right and left demonstrating parenchymal vascular supply to the
topographical lobar structure.

Despite Langenbuch's interest, in general, disorders of the liver did not command great attention in the closing days of the Nineteenth Century. Few patients
would present with external findings of liver enlargement, masses, or severe tender-
ness. Since diagnoses were most often made by careful physical examination—
visual inspection, touching, probing, pushing—few liver tumors could be felt,
tucked away as they were under the costal margin. Only those of enormous size or
literally hanging from the anterior liver surface would be detected. Most, unless
they produced systemic manifestations, went largely unnoticed until death and discovered only by autopsy. As a consequence, roughly half of his extensive textbook
would be taken up by discussions of liver abscesses and the other half on
Echinococcus disease, conditions often brought to light by painful swellings, fevers,
malaise, palpable and painful enlargement of the liver, and other systemic findings.

Hepatic echinococcus had been described by *Professeur* Joseph Récamier at the
Hôtel Dieu in Paris in 1825 as painful swellings of the liver—a type of hepatitis:

> The liver was very much enlarged; it descended more than two finger-steps below the rib
> borders, and extended as far as the epigastric region; its outer color was greenish brown; it
> was softened much more friable and easier to incise than it is in the state of health; it was
> filled with an immense number of small foci, the size of which ranged from pea to
> hazel … whose walls were devoid of internal membrane, [and] contained a homogeneous
> liquid of purulent consistency and a yellow color drawing a little on the green.

Récamier's treatment was simple—direct puncture and simple incision, empty-
ing cyst contents of an "aqueous and limpid liquid". Results were mixed [16]. The
eminent Parisian pathologist Gabriel Andral noted that opening of these cysts was
promptly followed by "fatal accidents" and that the operation was rejected by prudent surgeons [17]. Yet Récamier had reported a number of successes, provoking a
re-evaluation.

Decades after Récamier's description, the condition was graphically described
by Rudolf Virchow in Würzburg in 1855, presenting as a "gelatinous tumor of the
liver" containing pus-like fluid and, microscopically small alveolar vesicles, caused
by the larval stage of the tapeworm *Echinococcus multilocularis* [18, 19]. It was the
ingenious Russian surgeon Nikolai Sklifosovsky who, in 1887 reported three cases
of Echinococcal disease treated by, first, trocar aspiration of cyst contents, then
marsupalization of the cyst wall to the abdominal cavity, and finally, washing of the

---

⁵Carl Langenbuch, *Chirurgie der Leber und Gallenblase*, p 1; of note, Billroth's textbook of 1863
did not even mention diseases or surgery on the liver.

cyst lining with "corrosive sublimate". All three patients were reported cured of their affliction (see Ref. [20]; for a discussion of the life and works of this notable Russian surgeon see Ref. [21]). Similarly, the Argentinian Surgeon Alexandre Posadas had reported from Buenos Aires in 1899 his approach to surgery for hydatid disease by incising, draining, and then stripping the germinal membrane, thus eradicating parasitic tissue. "[A]fter the extraction of the germinal membrane and hydatid liquid, the walls of the peri-cystic pocket naturally come into contact, without the need for sutures." Posadas went on to say, thus closing the liver defect. This obviated the need for removal of large portions of the liver but with equivalent outcomes. Of 23 such cases of liver Echinococcus, in which this was attempted, recovery was seen in 19 and 4 (17%) died [22].

The Corsican surgeon Joseph-Antoine Pantaloni (1862–1909) who trained in Marseille and later wrote the expansive text *Chirurgie du Foie et des Voies Biliares* in 1899 was critical of those casual abdominal surgeons who assaulted the liver without proper preparation. Procedures on the liver, he cautioned, requires experience in visceral surgery and should be tried only by a surgeon who has proven expertise in gastrointestinal surgery. The danger lies chiefly, he stressed, in inadvertently removing too great a part of the organ; this can cause, if not serious functional disorders, at least enormous difficulties in hemostasis during the eradication of neoplasms. Specifically, with respect to hydatid cysts, "[a]t this time, the opening of these tumors [hydatid cysts] was formally condemned and it took audacity not to fear attacking them". Spilling of contents into the peritoneal cavity were met with spiraling sepsis and sometimes an untoward outcome [23].

But liver maladies frequently confronted the general surgeon. Hepatic abscesses were common in the Nineteenth Century. Professor Bärensprung of the *Berliner pathologischen Institutes* uncovered 108 cases among 7326 examined from the years 1859–1873. Langenbuch surmised that most of these were due to gallbladder pathology or some type of embolic phenomena from distant inflammatory disorders (see Ref. [15], p 201–202). Both were addressed by the requisite drainage (*Wo Eiter ist, verschaffe ihm Ausgang!* "Where there is pus, give it an exit!"), either by incision down to the cavity or by puncture (see Ref. [15], p 318). The surgical approach, Langenbuch described, was a challenging endeavor because of the "peculiar" location of the liver and its contained abscess that required particular demands of surgical skill and sometimes, if the swelling (*tumor* and *rubor*) is not immediately apparent, intimidates the probing surgeon until "his already raised hand sinks back undecided" (see Ref. [15], p 319). The constant threat, as might be expected, for Langenbuch was that dissection through liver parenchyma could be hazardous: *es riefe zu leicht lebensgefährliche Blutungen* "it caused, too easily, life-threatening bleeding" (see Ref. [15], p 327). Nowhere in this treatise does Langenbuch discuss removal of liver tissue other than in conjunction with infectious etiologies, and then, only in approaching the focus of pus. His peculiar liver resection of 1887 was not mentioned, so unorthodox he felt it to be.

References

1. Lincoln DF (1871) A Letter from Vienna, June 7, 1871. Boston Med Surg J 85:4–7
2. Lenoir T (1992) Laboratories, medicine and public life in Germany 1830-1849. In: Cunningham A, Williams P (eds) The laboratory revolution in medicine. Cambridge University Press, Cambridge, pp 14–71; quotes, 26, 35-36
3. Treves F (1900) Address in surgery: the surgeon of the nineteenth century. Brit Med J 2:284–289
4. von Bergmann E (1882) Die Gruppirung der Wundkrankheiten. Berliner klinische Wochenschrift 45:677–679
5. Senn N (1887) Lucerne, Berne and Geneva. JAMA 9:379–382
6. Billroth T (1863) Die allgemeine chirurgische Pathologie und Therapie. Georg Reimer, Berlin, p 14
7. Schlich T (2012) Asepsis and bacteriology: a realignment of surgery and laboratory science. Med Hist 56:308–334
8. Worboys M (2013) Joseph Lister and the performance of antiseptic surgery. Notes Rec R Soc 67:199–209
9. von Bergmann E (1882) Ueber antiseptische Wundbehandlung. Deutsche Medicinische Wochenschrift 43:571–572
10. Lesch JE (1984) Science and medicine in France: the emergence of experimental physiology, 1790–1855. Harvard University Press, Cambridge
11. Gluck T (1883) Ueber die Bedeutung physiologisch-chirurgischer Experimente an der Leber. Archiv fur Klinische Chirurgie 29:139–145
12. Kocher T (1890) Beitrage zur Chirurgie der Gallenwege. Dtsch Med Wochenschr 16:253–257
13. Langenbuch C (1882) Ein Fall von Exstirpation der Gallenblase wegen chronischer Cholelithiasis. Berliner klinische Wochenschrift 48:725–727
14. Langenbuch C (1888) Ein Fall von Resection eines Linksseitigen Schnurlappens der Leber. Berliner klinische Wochenschrift 25:37–38
15. Langenbuch C (1894) Chirurgie der Leber und Gallenblase. Ferdinand Enke, Stuttgart, p 1
16. Récamier J (1825) Des Maladies Observées a l'Hôtel-Dieu dans les Salles de Clinique de M. le Professeur Récamier, Pendant le Quatrieme Trimestre de 1824. Revue Médicale:1–54; including all listed quotes
17. Andral G (1839) Cours de Pathologie Interne. J.-B. Tircher, Brussels, p 262
18. Virchow R (1855) Die Multiloculaire Ulcerirende Echinokokkengeschwulst der Leber. Verhandlungen der Physicalisch-Medicinischen Gesellschaft Wurtzburg:84–95
19. Tappe DF (2007) Rudolf Virchow and the recognition of alveolar Echinococcosis, 1850s. Emerg Infect Dis 13:732–735
20. Sklifosovsky NV (1887) Operations for Echinococci of liver. Ann Surg 5:361–362
21. Kabanova SA (2016) N.V. Sklifosovsky—Creator of the clinical medicine campus in Devichye pole in Moscow (on the 180th anniversary of his birth). Hist Med 3:62–69
22. Posadas A (1899) Traitement des Kystes Hydatiques. Rev Chir 19:374–387
23. Pantaloni JA (1899) Chirurgie du Foie et des Voies Biliares. Institut de Bibliographie Scientifique, Paris, p 138

Chapter 5
Fin de Siècle: Marvels of the Age

Across the Atlantic surgery had entered a new era. "[T]he progress of surgery in the past twenty years is one of the marvels of the age. Anaesthetics [sic] and the outcome of antiseptics have stimulated the phenomenal development of this branch of medical sciences" so proclaimed Dr. Ernest Lewis in his presidential address before the Southern Surgical and Gynecological Association in 1896 [1]. And to that effect, American surgeon William Williams Keen (1837–1932), Professor of Surgery at the Jefferson Medical College in Philadelphia, had encountered a 53-year-old woman in February of 1897 who had noticed a tumor "at the pit of her stomach" 5 years ago. Keen was a well-educated physician, having attended Brown University as an undergraduate and Jefferson Medical College, graduating in 1862. However the year prior he had been sworn into the Army as assistant surgeon. Shortly thereafter he found himself near Manassas Creek for the first engagement of the American Civil War. "My experience in this battle," he later wrote, "is a good illustration of the utter disorganization … of our entire army at the beginning of the war" [2]. After his graduation from Jefferson in March 1862 (apparently a two-year course of study) Keen returned to military duty until the end of the war, caring for the horrible wounds, gangrene, and secondary hemorrhages that the times before antisepsis created.

Keen then had spent time in Europe, visiting the *Allgemeine Krankenhaus* in Vienna in 1865. "A magnificent place to learn" he had written to acquaintances in the United States, although he was appalled at the impersonal treatment many of these patients endured as they were shuffled in front of a gawking, spell-bound audience [3]. Now, his patient had recently begun having severe abdominal pain, presumably from the tumor. It was clearly palpable to Keen and although he was not certain of the etiology determined that an operation was needed. This would not be his first venture into the liver. Not known for his temerity nor lacking in self-confidence, on October 9, 1891, he had operated on a young woman, 31 years old, for a palpable tumor, initially the size of a walnut but with her pregnancy it had enlarged to the size of a fist, by the time Keen examined her. "Until ten years ago

T. S. Helling, D. Azoulay, *Historical Foundations of Liver Surgery*,
https://doi.org/10.1007/978-3-030-47095-1_5

the liver was not deemed amenable to surgical attack on account of its vascularity," he prefaced. Yet, confident of being able to check the hemorrhage, he proceeded. On opening the abdomen Keen encountered the tumor attached to the lateral edge of her liver. He had then performed a wedge-type excision using his Paquelin's cautery

> I tried the effect of the Paquelin cautery, and was so well satisfied with it that I made no further attempt to ligate the liver-substance but continued cutting with the cautery. As I cut, four very large veins were laid bare, and were ligated before being burned through

As the tumor extended into the substance of the liver, Keen then stripped "the liver-substance from the tumor with my thumb-nail, and found that I could do so with perfect ease and without serious haemorrhage." He then approximated the two edges of the liver together with five sutures. The tumor proved to be a cystic adenoma and the patient recovered [4].

So here would be his second case of liver resection. On March 4, 1897, with William Coplin, Professor of Pathology at Jefferson, in attendance, Keen entered the woman's abdomen via a right paramedian incision. He found a 7.5 cm pedunculated tumor located "just to the left of the notch where the round ligament was attached," in today's terminology, segment III. The surgeons agreed that it looked like an angioma. Keen was leery of a direct "attack" with knife or cautery and, by cutting down on some liver tissue, formed a "pedicle" which he ligated with elastic rubber tubes. The abdomen was partially closed with the tumor protruding. The tumor was inspected at 48 h and "was distinctly shrinking and showed signs of strangulation." By day six the rubber ligatures were removed. There was a small pedicle remaining which was snipped with scissors, removing the tumor, "without the loss of a drop of blood." She recovered uneventfully. The tumor was, on inspection by Coplin, indeed, an (hem)angioma [5].

Emboldened by his first two successes, on April 23, 1899, Keen embarked on his third case, found to be a large 14 × 11 × 7 cm tumor occupying the topographical left lobe of a 50-year-old clothing inspector. In contrast to his first two cases where there was more or less a liver pedicle or liver edge that could be treated as a "stalk" away from major vessels, this case would entail transection of liver all the way to the hepatic veins. Using Paquelin's cautery almost entirely, he slowly burned his way through liver substance, needing to ligate five large veins with catgut suture threaded onto a large Hagedorn needle. Once the tumor was removed, as he had done before, he folded the edges of the liver together and secured them with suture. As a precaution against delayed bleeding he then stuffed iodoform gauze against the liver and brought the end out through the wound as a sort of drain. He estimated his blood loss at about 300 mL. The patient had an uneventful recovery, and the iodoform gauze was removed after 48 h. There was minimal bile leak after that, in total about 120 mL. The tumor proved to be a carcinoma [6].

For his third case Keen may have been influenced by the writings of Russians Michel Kousnetzoff and Jules Pensky, both Associate Professors of Surgery at Kharkov University in the Ukraine, who published in 1896 an extensive review of their experiments on liver resection in dogs, rabbits, and human cadavers [7]. Their work focused on controlling hemorrhage through the application of tamponade, including placement of iodoform gauze in the liver wound and suturing over it, as well as the application of omentum to the raw liver surface. In addition, they introduced the practice of placing a continuous mattress suture above the resection line, feeling that mass ligature, gently done, was preferable to isolation and ligation of individual structures that often resulted in tearing of their lateral branches. They stressed delicacy in handling liver vessels, although at the same time pointing out the durability of portal pedicles, enveloped in Glisson's thick connective tissue as they coursed through liver substance. Incorporation of portal pedicles, careful handling of hepatic venous structures, and application of pressure would become lasting principles of hepatic surgery.

The remarkable hemostatic device that Keen so fondly embraced, Paquelin's cautery, was invention of Claude-André Paquelin (1836–1905) (Figs. 5.1 and 5.2). It was a thermocautery consisting of a glass bottle filled with petroleum ether. The attached bulb was used to squeeze vapor from the bottle through a rubber tube to the instrument's heated platinum tip where it was ignited, thus providing cauterization, essentially a handheld blow torch. It was easy to use, and relatively effective yet quite expensive because of the platinum tip. Of course there was some danger to the

Fig. 5.1 Wiilliam Keen (1837–1932) ©The National Library of Medicine

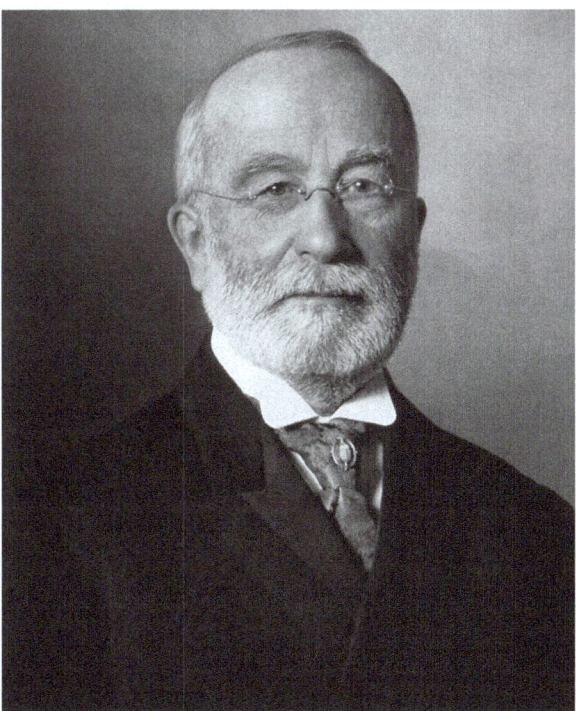

Fig. 5.2 Paquelin's cautery. From Frank Foster, an illustrated encyclopaedic medical dictionary, 1890. ©The National Library of Medicine

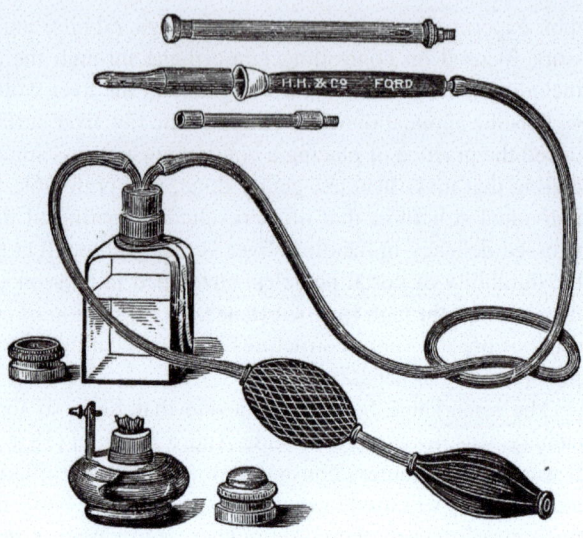

operator if the bottle caught fire [8]. For those who could afford it, the cautery evidently added some degree of hemostasis to the cut liver surface.[1]

By 1899 Keen had compiled a total of 76 cases of liver resection including 17 of his own patients. All must have presented as a palpable mass below the right subcostal margin, many it seems had been present for years. Of 74 verifiable cases, he could determine that there had been 11 deaths, a mortality rate of 15%. Most cases, of course, were individual reports from centers in Europe. And most, from Keen's descriptions, were pedunculated as judged by the major concern of the operating surgeons as to how the "stump" should be treated. Many of these amputated bases had stopped bleeding and were merely returned to the abdominal cavity; some were stitched to the wound and packed with iodoform gauze or other caustic substances [6]. Hemorrhage continued to be the major threat to liver surgery. In Keen's mind, this was the key to a successful outcome: sealing the cut surface of the liver. While some vessels were sturdy (enveloped by Glisson's capsule), others were quite flimsy and held sutures poorly. A combination of tamponade and suturing seemed to eventually produce hemostasis if the surgeon was patient, gentle, and meticulous.

Keen wrote extensively about the liver and its surgical conditions. He devoted considerable space to it in his 1899 textbook of surgery. Like Langenbuch his primary focus was on echinococcal disease and liver abscesses. For abscesses the surgical approach was familiar: wide exposure, needle localization of the abscess, fixing the liver to the abdominal wall, opening down to the abscess, drainage, and

---

[1] Paquelin's device was first presented in 1876 to *l'Académie des Sciences* in Paris [9]. Actually, an "electric cautery" had been introduced in France by Joseph Charrière (1803–1876), manufacturer of *instruments de chirurgie* in 1855. American physician observers in Paris at that time noted that by using the electric apparatus "the desired result can be obtained without shocking the non-professional observer by the horrible sight of 'red-hot pokers'" [10].

irrigation. As for the occasional liver neoplasm, Keen felt such conditions were not surgical in nature. "Carcinoma, sarcoma, gumma, lymphoma, adenoma, and erectile tumors are seen in the liver, but usually they are not amenable to surgical treatment." Keen also made mention of anecdotal work done on liver resection, particularly, Langenbuch's encounter with the corseted lady and attempts to excise portions of liver involved with Echinococcal disease. Useful instruments, he mentioned, were the knife, thermo-cautery, and elastic ligatures. His only commentary on the vascular nature of liver substance? "Free hemorrhage sometimes occurs in operating on the liver, which is usually rapidly arrested by tamponing [sic] with iodoform gauze and securing the bleeding vessels" [11].[2]

Keen's fame spread internationally. He received accolades from the great Theodor Kocher of Bern, Switzerland, in his 1907 textbook *Chirurgische Operationslehre*. Kocher acknowledged Keen's prowess in resecting liver tumors "with a happy result" and echoed Keen's enthusiasm about the future of liver surgery ("Keen … has become very confident about the prospects of this operation"), largely based on Keen's compilation of 76 cases with only a 15% mortality. Kocher then waxed philosophically about proper techniques of dividing "soft" liver parenchyma, as "exhausting" hemorrhage was often an untoward result. How to stem the bleeding? He recommended the use of Paquelin's thermo-cautery as Keen had employed, and suggested mass ligatures reinforced by strips of iodoform gauze soaked in carbolic acid (Figs. 5.3 and 5.4). Kocher even proposed the use of a broad curved intestinal clamp—*große und fest zu schließende* (large and tight-fitting)—that he often employed for gastroenterostomies—to be applied to the cut surface of the liver. In fact, Kocher would leave the clamps in place—even on the thick right lobe—protruding out of the abdominal incision for days, allowing for eventual hemostasis of the cut surfaces. With such an open wound one might wonder, of course, about the prospects of evisceration in the meantime. In fact, Keen himself had reported two such cases employing these clamps—neither one done by Kocher—in his 1899 review. One died and one survived. Despite such bravado, most liver resections continued to be wedge-shaped affairs close to the liver's anterior edge [6, 12].

William Keen went on to become most famous for his work in neurologic surgery, writing extensively on neuroanatomy and neurophysiology, and, along with Harvey Cushing and Walter Dandy, perfecting techniques of brain surgery. Because of the scope of his interests he would be anointed one of the three "Marshalls" of American surgery aside his contemporaries William Halsted and Cushing (the eminent Samuel D. Gross was crowned the "Emperor"). Despite producing hundreds of article, books, and editorials, he wrote no more on surgery of the liver. Yet his demeanor and comportment set the stage for all future liver surgeons working with an organ so volatile. According to his assistant and eventual successor at Jefferson, John Chalmers DaCosta, "He always showed best when the situation was worst. Dr.

---

[2] Including all quotes; this was the first American surgery text based on Listerian principles.

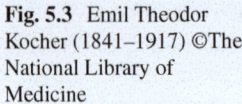

Fig. 5.3 Emil Theodor
Kocher (1841–1917) ©The
National Library of
Medicine

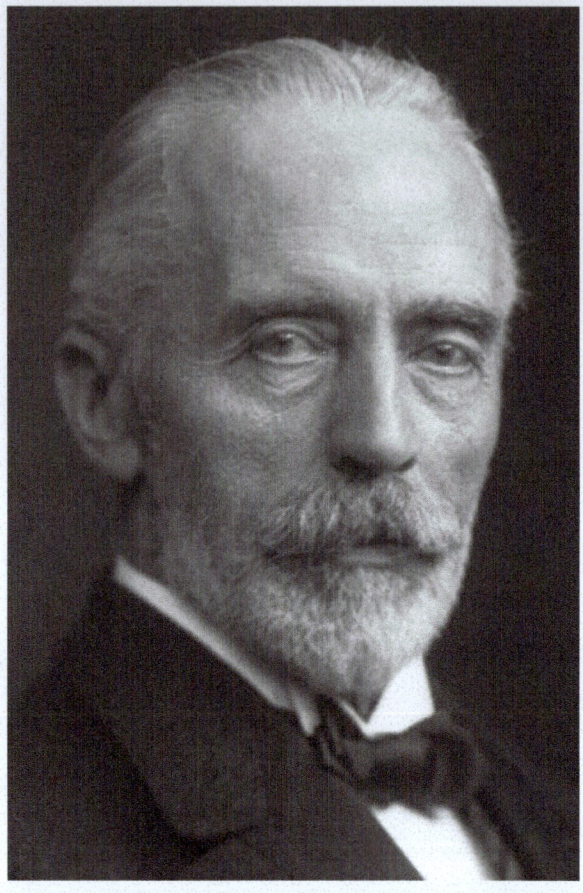

Keen was always, calmer, quieter, kinder, pleasanter, the worse the surgical situation was, and I never saw it get the best of him." [13].

Whether Keen was the first to perform a liver resection in the United States is arguable. Louis McLane Tiffany (1844–1916), Professor of Surgery at the University of Maryland, reported, in brief, the removal of a portion of the left lobe of the liver through a five-inch left paramedian incision in a 25-year-old farmer in 1890, predating Keen's work by a year. Tiffany's patient likely suffered from biliary calculus disease [14].[3] The ambidextrous surgeon removed the tumor from the convex surface of the liver (from symptomatology, meaning the left "lobe") with curved scissors and obtained hemostasis with cautery, leaving a liver cavity "the size of a walnut." All seemed to go well, the patient recuperating 18 days later, at the time of his presentation. The prior month, before the American Surgical Association in

---

[3] Tiffany reported his case before the 236th meeting of the Clinical Society of Maryland June 6, 1890.

Fig. 5.4 Kocher's technique of applying strips of iodoform gauze soaked in carbolic acid to the cut liver edges secured by mattress sutures. Chirurgische Operationslehre, 1907, p. 832

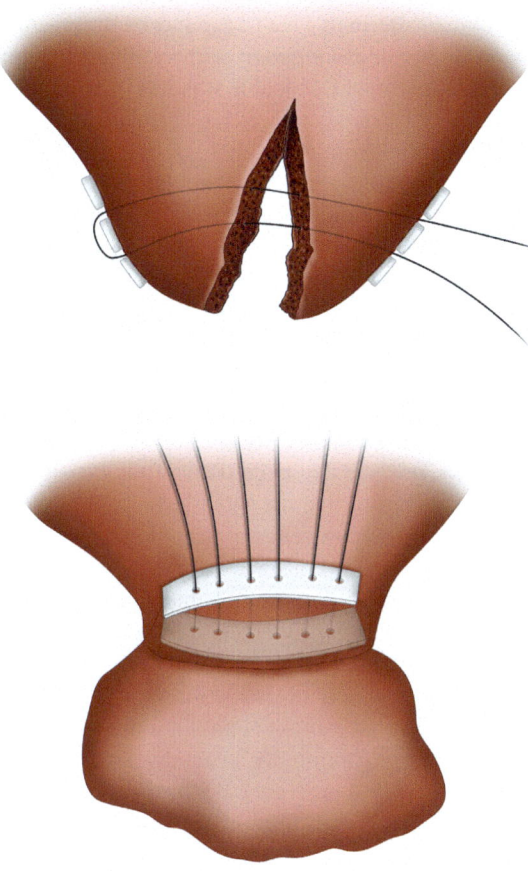

Washington, DC, Tiffany had presented his principles of liver surgery, perhaps based on his one recent case, emphasizing that "surgery of the liver is to be considered as is the surgery of the rest of the body, not as surgery apart from everything else." Bleeding and bile leak, he claimed, were within the skills of surgeons to confront, and healing could be induced "by appropriate treatment." In short, basic surgical techniques—patience, gentleness, diligence—apply to any anatomic structure. The liver was no different [15]. One might imagine Tiffany's informal manner in illuminating his philosophy, casually leaning on the amphitheater railing as he often did in lecturing, almost as if he were conversing about the weather. His personality was warming, his demeanor self-effacing, yet his accomplishments irrefutable.

In Germany anecdotal experiences continued. The rarity of liver tumors meant that no vast experience by any one surgeons would accumulate—and each, because of the anxieties of surgical extirpation, was duly examined and published. Prior to 1900 no less than 15 surgeons had reported their individual cases in the literature. Typical of those descriptions was that of the great Ernst von Bergmann (1836–1907), the distinguished Professor of Surgery at the University of Berlin and successor to the famous Bernard von Langenbeck. Bergmann had encountered a 61-year-old man who became alarmed by with swelling in the upper abdomen and a lump which he could easily feel. Palpable was a mobile tumor "the size of a child's head" with a smooth consistency suggestive of a hydatid cyst. Bergmann operated with an incision extending from the xiphoid process to the navel. The tumor was immediately obvious, seemingly arising from the left lobe, gray-red in appearance. He deftly eviscerated the tumor-bearing liver, the tumor itself attached to the liver by a broad pedicle 12 wide and 2 cm thick. Transhepatic sutures did not hold, perhaps placed too close to the edge. Bergmann quickly used his assistant's fingers to compress liver substance as he cut a short distance, found individual vessels, and ligated them "a procedure that was painful and time-consuming, for here, too, the ligatures tore through." Even after that "blood seeped quite vividly from various places." It was then that he used Paquelin's thermocautery to touch up any bleeding points. Caustic iodoform gauze was thickly applied to the raw surface, and Bergmann let the liver sink back into the abdomen. Part of his incision he left open to expose the gauze impregnated operative site and—he had used this method for many intestinal operations—to allow slow removal of the gauze later. Delayed bleeding was a notorious event, commanding constant surveillance of the open wound and a prompt decision to explore should evidence of hemorrhage present. Bergmann's tumor proved to be that mixture of cellular elements characteristic of a hepatic adenoma. One year later the patient was fully recovered. There was no evidence of recurrence and the wound itself had completely healed [16].

Indeed Joseph-Antoine Pantaloni had good reason to admonish the occasional liver surgeon. "Admittedly," Pantaloni wrote, "the operative methods are improving every day and push back the limits of these procedures; but it is prudent not to dare, especially with tumors not pedunculated [*i.e.* within the substance of the liver]" [17]. Such adventures should only be done with a firm grasp on how exposure, mobilization, and hemostasis would be achieved, he cautioned. In this regard, Pantaloni outlined a certain number of steps, common in all cases, deduced from the numerous observations published (and quite familiar to hepatic surgeons of today): (1) careful examination of the "sick part" at the beginning of the exploratory laparotomy; (2) the mobilization and externalization of the diseased portion as much as possible; (3) the mode of attack of the lesion with the ability to control hemostasis *before* parenchymal dissection (placement of broad parenchymal sutures through liver substance) and the availability of "special instruments" such as thermocautery—Pantaloni argued that scalpel sectioning was most efficient for intra-parenchymal tumors, although the surgeon should be at the ready to effect hemostasis; and (4) familiarity with different methods used to obtain absolute hemostasis of the hepatic pedicle such as thermocautery, tamponade, suture ligatures for individual bleeding points, or even ligation of major hepatic vessels (Fig. 5.5).

Yet accidents of various kinds have been noted, Pantaloni warned. Of course, one of the most serious was delayed hemorrhage. One should not hesitate, in those situations, to reopen the abdomen for control, he emphasized. Another that was brought

Fig. 5.5 A diagram of Joseph-Antoine Pantaloni's laparotomy incisions for access to the liver. From Pantaloni, in Chirurgie du foie et des voies biliaires, 1899

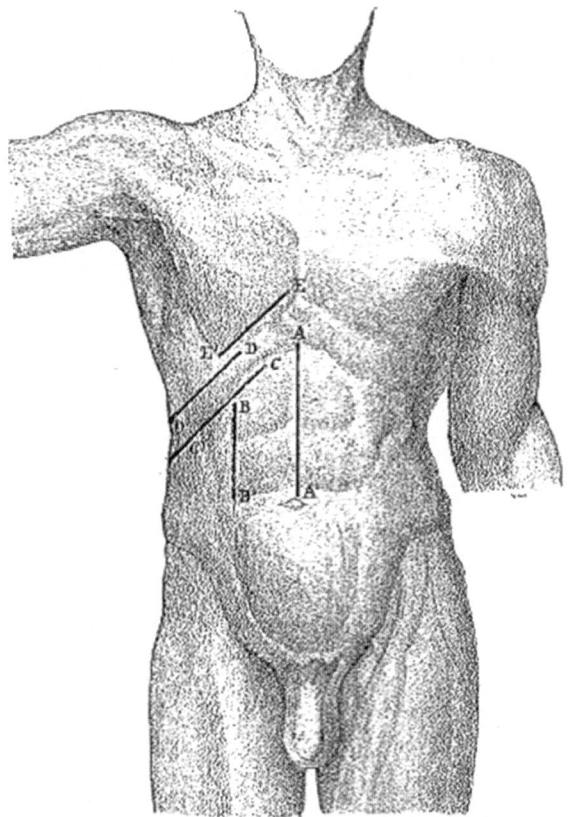

to his attention was a case of profuse venous bleeding requiring tamponade. The patient died 2 h later from what was recognized at autopsy as a "gas [air] embolism" (see [17], 164–175).

Pantaloni was not alone in his trepidations. The third urban general hospital for the city of Berlin, *der Krankenhause am Urban* opened in 1889 with 570 beds. The hospital was "fitted up in accordance with the most advanced modern ideas as to hygienic requirements and the comfort of patients."[4] To direct the surgical department young Professor Werner Körte (1853–1937) was named. His interest in liver and gallbladder surgery prompted publishing a textbook *Beiträge zur Chirurgie der Gallenwege und der Leber* in 1905. Just as with Langenbuch's textbook on liver surgery Körte focused on infectious diseases affecting the liver, namely, liver abscesses. Neoplasms occupied much less space. Like Keen, Körte felt solid tumors were not a surgical disease. "Benign tumors of the liver are rare … and malignant tumors are metastatic in nature … and thus usually unsuitable for operation." However, if surgery is contemplated, he opined, resection is greatly facilitated if a

---

[4] British Medical Journal, June 28, 1890, p. 1521 (no author).

pedicle is present or if the neoplasm lies on the edge of the liver substance. Digital compression, elastic bands, or clips he recommended for hemostasis and to prevent air ingress to "gaping hepatic veins." Körte used long blunt-tipped needles threaded with catgut suture to penetrate liver substance and control bleeding (tied very carefully as "the consistency of the liver tissue is exceedingly different, with some livers so soft that you cannot create a durable seam"). He warned against diving too deep into liver substance. In those depths "bleeding is uncertain, therefore, the extirpation of such located tumors is not recommended" [18].

Yet by the close of the nineteenth century European surgeons had accumulated enough experience dealing with liver wounds and liver surgery that certain precepts were developed and commonly discussed. Elective resections of hepatic neoplasms remained an infrequent occurrence, however. "We must first recognize that tumor cases in which the surgeon is allowed to intervene must be considered as very rare," began Louis-Félix Terrier (1837–1908) in his 1901 treatise *Chirurgie du Foie et des Voies biliares*. Like his contemporaries, Terrier understood the benefit of a stalk or pedicle of liver tissue from which a tumorous lesion seemed to arise. He called this "*pediculisation*"—"pediculization." With a stalk, Terrier reckoned, the entire base could be externalized, encircled, and compressed for control of bleeding once the tumor had been excised. Indeed, in the days before radiography, most palpable tumors arose from liver edge and would, of course, have a manageable base of liver substance, the sought after "pedicle." "There can be no question," Terrier went on, "about tackling tumors deep in the thickness of the organ, for reasons which are unnecessary to mention [hemorrhage]." This was why the wise surgeons would be loath to resect without the desired pedicle [19]. And for hemorrhage and the ensuing "commotion"? Terrier hoped the patient was "robust with a strong constitution." Stimulants such as alcohol, ether, ammonia, rest, and opium could be tried. Or, in extreme cases, bleeding—both locally over the liver (by scarified cupping) and from the extremities by venesection—was even suggested (although its efficacious manner was never fully explained). None of the hemostatic means should be neglected, not even bleeding "to the point of mellowing the almost bloodless patient."[5] Combing the literature, Terrier was able to produce 52 cases of curative resection for liver tumors (including hydatid disease and syphilitic gumma) with 10 deaths, a mortality of 19 percent. While acknowledging that shock, sepsis, and hemorrhage were the principle causes of death, and despite his dire warnings of near-fatal bleeding, he was surprised to learn that hemorrhage was responsible for only two of the 10 deaths (shock cases were almost certainly hemorrhagic in origin, however):

> The hemorrhage was hitherto the great complication to be dreaded, and it may be surprising that, even in the absence of a good operative technique, it has not been observed more often; indeed, we find it reported only twice in our observations (see [19], p 242).

---

[5] This was a technique to counter voluminous liver bleeding from trauma advocated by Félix Marie Gabriel Roustan (1849–1885) in his 1875 text *Des Lesions Traumatiques du Foie* (Paris: Adrien Delahaye, 1875); quotes taken from Roustan, 118.

A fellow countryman, the notoriously flamboyant French surgeon Eugène-Louis Doyen (1859–1916), popularized the technique of pedicle ligation and either excising or simply waiting for the strangulated liver tumor to literally fall off. Otherwise, with good hemostasis, the liver stump was returned to the abdominal cavity and, contrary to the practices of German surgeon von Bergmann, the incision fully closed. While hydatid disease was a primary focus, the engaging Doyen boldly claimed that "almost all liver pathology now belongs to the surgeon," insisting that surgeons now "must never neglect the exploration of the total liver, under pain of exposing ourselves to serious mischief" [20].

Doyen echoed sentiments shared by many of his contemporaries. By 1900 surgeons felt the liver was well within their scope of practice, if only hemostasis could be assured. Ingenious methods were found. Two Italians, Andrea Ceccherelli and Angelo Bianchi, proposed using very thin slices of decalcified and softened whalebone as buttresses on either side of the liver pedicle much as today's pledgets are used. These whalebone buttresses would eventually absorb [21]. The Genoan Giovanni Segale, presenting at the 13th *Congrès International de Médecine* held in Paris in 1900, modified this approach by using small pegs (*chevilles*) of ivory or ebonite through which catgut suture was threaded (Fig. 5.6). Placed on either side of the liver substance the two bars of pegs were then approximated with elastic threads that cause compression of the liver and hemostasis. The desired liver portion was then excised and the two bars of pegs were encapsulated and remain innocuous to the host [22]. This method was employed by French surgeons and duly described by Terrier in his textbook of liver surgery. In fact, Terrier, experimenting on the dog liver, developed a technique for the intrahepatic control of major blood vessels via a large curved needle on which could be passed large suture from the superior liver surface to the inferior surface. Tying these "by tightening with slow and continuous traction" seemed to control those vessels feeding the liver portion to be removed (see [19], p 213–216).

Wilhelm "Willy" Anschütz (1870–1954) was a pupil and assistant to the great surgeon Johann von Mikulicz (1850–1905) in Wroclaw (Breslau) Poland. It was

Fig. 5.6 The procedure of Giovanni Segale using pegs of ivory through which catgut suture was passed to provide hemostasis for the cut liver surface. From Terrier, in Chirurgie du Foie et des Voies Biliares, 1901

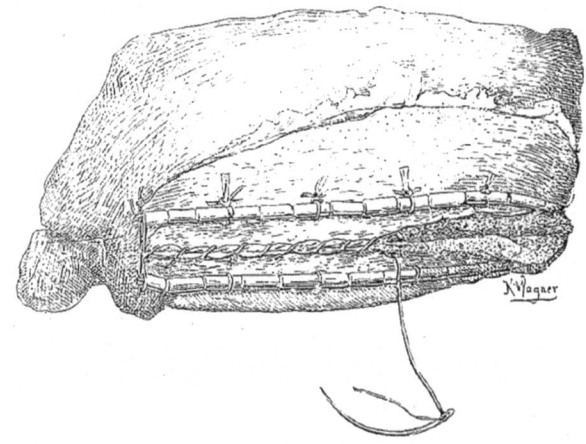

there that he developed an interest in surgery of the liver and also courted and wed Hilda von Mikulicz, the eldest daughter of his mentor. In 1903, he compiled and published a treatise entitled *Über die Resection der Leber* ("About Resection of the Liver"). In this publication he reviewed 90 liver operations up to 1903 according to the method of dealing with the "liver stump" performed by 70 different surgeons. No surgeon performed more than six operations (Johann Mikulicz did six, Ernesto Tricomi six and Vincenz Czerny four) and 61 performed only one. Overall there were 21 deaths (23%). Highest mortality was seen after "tamponade and compression" (44%) and use of intraparenchymal ligatures (36%), but this may have simply reflected the larger extent of the liver resection. With simple suture closure of the raw cut surface only one of 25 expired. As for the infrequency of this type of surgery, Anschütz fully realized it was well within the purview of the competent visceral surgeon and that

> [E]ven if we rarely have the opportunity to practice the technique of liver resection on humans, we should not be reluctant to review them from time to time, in order to be prepared for any dangers threatening the success of liver resections

Included in Anschütz's series was another case (or perhaps the same case as reported by Pantaloni) of air embolism. Julius Hochenegg (1859–1940), surgeon and protégé of Theodor Billroth, described an unfortunate patient he encountered in 1898. A 57-year-old man had undergone removal of a large "adenoma" very close to a large hepatic vein. Soon rapid bleeding occurred from the depth of the liver wound controlled by compression, but the patient could not be saved and expired on the operating table. The autopsy reviewed air emboli in the heart [23].

German ingenuity, driven by the commanding influence of Theodor Billroth, continued. Professor Walther Wendel (1872–1941) succeeded the esteemed Professor Rudolf Habs (1863–1937), a former understudy of Mikulicz and Billroth, as chief surgeon at the hospital in the medieval city of Magdeburg-Sudenburg.[6] In an unassuming stroke of daring he was to expand the potential of liver surgery. His prompt was a frail, depressed, 44-year-old woman who had suffered from hemorrhage first recognized during her last pregnancy, causing extreme debilitation and leaving her exhausted. A *"blasse, sehr elende, magere Frau"*—a pale, very miserable, skinny woman—was she, weighing a mere 45 kg. Most notable in this scaphoid abdomen was an obviously enlarged right lobe of her liver, visible and easily palpated below the right costal margin. Because of the rapid enlargement of her liver Wendel worried that this indeed was a liver neoplasm, either primary or secondary. On July 18, 1910, he operated. A midline incision was used with a right extension into the upper abdomen, thus exposing the entire liver. The left liver lobe, gallbladder, and liver hilum appeared normal but the right lobe was occupied by a

---

[6]Rudolf Habs was a local celebrity. He received his surgical training in Magdeburg and returned there after his fellowships in Wrocław (modern Breslau), the Prussian home to Mikulicz, and Vienna. He was the first chief surgeon at the new surgical department at the Hospital Magdeburg-Sudenburg, achieving fame in abdominal and orthopedic surgery. Wendel studied for 10 years under Ernst Kuster at the University Hospital in Marburg and was appointed associate professor in 1905. The following year he moved to Magdeburg-Sudenburg Hospital.

doppeltfaustgrossen—double-fisted—tumor. He mobilized the right liver by dividing the coronary ligament and scooping the posterior liver and tumor from the retroperitoneum.[7] He then divided the right hepatic artery and right bile duct. The
portal vein was controlled, not at the hilum, for fear of clot propagation into the left
portal system, but by a series of intrahepatic ligatures of heavy catgut sutures passed
through the liver substance with an eyed, blunt-tipped needle based on principles
demonstrated by Kousnetzoff and Pensky. The right lobe was then divided with a
knife, leaving a 1 cm margin from the intrahepatic ligatures, in an almost bloodless
fashion. Bleeding that did occur was controlled with the familiar iodoform-soaked
gauze. Interestingly the gallbladder was left in place even though the cystic artery
was ligated and divided. It is difficult to tell for certain how much of this woman's
liver was removed. Likely, with retention of the gallbladder the resection plane may
have unknowingly traversed what would eventually be known as Cantlie's line,
although there is no specific reference to it or Cantlie in Wendel's article. The entire
specimen weighed 940 g. If one considers that liver weight is 2% of total body
weight, this woman's liver (0.02 × 45 kg) should have weighed 900 g. Half of her
liver (or more) plus weight of the large tumor would closely approximate 940 g.
Indeed, Wendel very well may have performed the first right hepatic lobectomy.

Despite her frailty, his subject weathered her ordeal, not even experiencing the
expected bile leak. Her tumor was diagnosed as a right-sided hepatic adenoma.
Almost 1 year later the woman, restored to health, weighed 63 kg. With her gain in
weight and sense of well-being, Wendel claimed complete victory. He later commented *"die fruheren nervosen beschwerden verschwunden"*—the earlier nervous
disorders have disappeared [24].[8]

Yet these anecdotal tales of surgical audacity did not dispel the real dangers of
such adventures and failed to convince many surgeons of the utility of hepatic resection. Uncontrollable hemorrhage and the fear of a death on the operating table gave
most surgeons a well-deserved pause. Certainly not all agreed with the illustrious
Eugène-Louis Doyen. For many the liver remained outside their realm of surgical
assaults. In the United States, at the 1912 meeting of the American Surgical
Association John McDill of Milwaukee rose to make the following observation:

> [I]t can still be said that surgery of the liver is an imperfectly developed field. From the
> beginning liver surgery has been feared and shunned on account of hemorrhage, and today
> notwithstanding the numerous and ingenious methods of hemostasis devised [26].[9]

---

[7] He thus described two enduring principles of liver surgery: wide exposure and complete mobilization. Only then can compression ("tamponade") be used as an adjunct in reducing bleeding
during parenchymal forays.

[8] Wendel achieved notoriety in esophageal and adrenal surgery but did not appear to broaden his
involvement in liver surgery by any additional publications. This woman was reported by Martin
Tinker to have suffered from primary adenocarcinoma of the liver. Tinker claims she died in 1919
and that an autopsy demonstrated extensive tumor recurrence [25].

[9] McDill later published a portion of this presentation in *Annals of Surgery* [27]. John Rich McDill
(1861–1934) had a long and distinguished career in the United States Army, serving in the
Philippines and also with the American Expeditionary Force in France during World War I. He also
held faculty appointments at Rush Medical College and the University of Chicago.

Yes, hemorrhage was indeed the curse of the liver surgeon. For as many as advocated righteous incursions, there were those who preached caution. The eminent Swiss surgeon Carl Garrè (1857–1928), student of the great Theodor Kocher, echoed the sentiments of many surgeons that in surgery of the liver "hemostasis presents the greatest difficulties." In 1907, he had commented to an American audience:

> Not much is to be expected from preventative hemostasis in the liver. As soon as the operation has advanced from the edge to the central portions of the liver, it is hardly possible to apply clamps which compress the bulky liver sufficiently to secure a bloodless operation [28].

In fact Garrè went on to say that "temporary ligation of the portal vein [to produce preventive hemostasis] cannot be accepted without grave objection" [28].

James Hogarth Pringle (1863–1941) would change all that. Pringle was born in Parramatta, New South Wales, Australia, a working suburb of Sidney, to George Hogarth and Annie Oakes Pringle. His father George (1830–1872), also a surgeon and close friend of Joseph Lister, introduced aseptic surgery to Australia. James received his medical education, not in Australia, but half a world away in Edinburgh, Scotland. He was then house surgeon to the Regius Chair of Surgery, Thomas Annandale (1838–1907), successor to Joseph Lister at Edinburgh. As did many surgeons-in-training of the day, James matriculated among the surgery centers of Europe (Berlin, Vienna, Hamburg), finally settling back in Scotland at the Royal Infirmary in Glasgow under tutelage of the peerless Scot Sir William Macewen (1848–1924) who commanded the title of Professor of Surgery at the University of Glasgow, a position also formerly held by his mentor, Joseph Lister. Pringle's father's connections to Lister and Glasgow possibly facilitated this posting for his son. Pringle became the consummate general surgeon but with leanings towards trauma and orthopedic surgery. It was with his passion for trauma that Pringle would make a singular contribution to liver surgery [29].

In a paper published in *Annals of Surgery* in 1908 Pringle described his experiences with liver trauma and the exsanguinating hemorrhage which took the lives of four of his patients. He noticed, though, during his surgery that pinching the portal vein and hepatic artery "completely arrested all bleeding." Unfortunately, despite this maneuver and the use of broad transhepatic ligatures as described by Kousnetzoff and Pensky, his patients soon died. However, he was impressed by the reduction in liver bleeding effected by controlling portal vein vessels [30]. That had not formerly been the experience of his contemporaries, besides Carl Garrè, Carl Langenbuch, and Emil Ponfick. In fact, Langenbuch and the German pathologist Emil Ponfick (1844–1913) had reported disastrous results from portal vein clamping in experimental animals and attributed the resultant vascular collapse to venous congestion of the splanchnic circulation and had suggested a rather elaborate process of compressing mesenteric veins in anticipation of portal vein occlusion—altogether an unsatisfactory arrangement, at least in the laboratory [31]. Pringle did not witness this vascular collapse in his patients and began to doubt the validity of their arguments, at least in humans. His observations led him to believe that ligation of the mesenteric arteries was time-wasting and unnecessary and that temporary portal obstruction could safely be done to reduce liver bleeding. In so doing he established an important principle of liver surgery—inflow occlusion as a preventative strategy in controlling bleeding during the parenchymal dissection in liver surgery. His technique would forever be known as the Pringle maneuver. In fact, by 1912, use of portal compression to facilitate bloodless liver surgery was advocated by others. Doctor John McDill had included his specially designed "enterostomy clamp" fitted with rubber tubing as useful in clamping across the hepatoduodenal ligament, compressing all portal inflow, in dogs for up to 30 min. It was a method, McDill optimistically claimed, that produced "bloodless surgery." However, McDill cautioned that he had observed (in his dogs) an ominous discoloration of the intestines, indicating a dangerous degree of back pressure [26].

References

1. Lewis ES (1897) The President's address. Trans Southern Surg Gynecol Assoc 9:1–8
2. Keen WW (1905) Surgical reminiscences of the civil war. Trans Coll Phys Philadelphia 27:95–114
3. Warner JH (1998) Against the spirit of system. Johns Hopkins University Press, Baltimore, p 304
4. Keen WW (1892) On resection of the liver, especially for hepatic tumors. Boston Med Surg J 126:405–409
5. Keen WW (1897) Removal of an angioma of the liver by elastic constriction external to the abdominal cavity, with a table of 59 cases of operation for hepatic tumors. Pennsylvania Med J 1:193–204
6. Keen WW (1899) Report of a case of resection of the liver for the removal of a neoplasm with a table of seventy-six cases of resection of the liver for hepatic tumors. Ann Surg 30:267–283
7. Kousnetzoff M, Pensky J (1896) Sur la Resection Partielle du Foie. Rev Chir 16:954–992
8. Tillmanns H (1901) A textbook of surgery. Appleton and Company, New York, pp 79–80
9. Paquelin C-A (1876) Sur un Nouveau Thermo-Cautere. Compt rendus seances de l'Academie des Sciences 82:1070
10. Suckley G (1858) Notes on the practice in the hospitals of Paris: the "Ecraseur", "electric cautery", Maisonneuve's method of diviving strictures, etc. Atlanta Med Surg J 3:656–670
11. Keen WW, White JW (1899) An American text-book of surgery for practitioners and students. W.B. Saunders, Philadelphia, pp 780–784
12. Kocher T (1907) Chirurgische Operationslehre. Jena, Gustav Fischer, pp 829–833, quotes 831, 832
13. Wagner FB (1989) Thomas Jefferson University: tradition and heritage. Lea & Febiger, Philadelphia, p 539
14. Tiffany LM (1890) The removal of a solid tumor from the liver by laparotomy. Maryland Med J 23:531
15. Tiffany LM (1890) Surgery of the liver. Boston Med Surg J 23:557
16. von Bergmann E (1893) Zur Cauistik der Leber-Chirurgie. Verhandlungen der Deutschen Gesellschaft fur Chirurgie, 22nd congress. Berlin, August Hirschwald, pp 218–238
17. Pantaloni JA (1899) Chirurgie du Foie et des Voies Biliares. Institut de Bibliographie Scientifique, Paris, p 184
18. Körte W (1905) Beiträge zur Chirurgie der Gallenwege und der Leber. August Hirschwald, Berlin, pp 261–267
19. Terrier F (1901) Chirurgie du Foie et des Voies Biliares. Felix Alcan, Paris, 32, 199

20. Doyen E (1892) Quelques Operations sur le Foie et les Voies Biliares. Arch Provinc Chir 1:149–178
21. Ceccherelli AB (1894) Nuovo Processo di Sutura per l'Emostasi del Fegato. Atti d. Cong. Med Internaz Sez Chir 4:188–191
22. Segale G (1900) Nouveau Procede pour l'Hemostase du Foie au Moyen d'une Suture Speciale Enchevillee. XIIIe Congrès International de Médecine. Masson, Paris, pp 254–259
23. Anschütz W (1903) Uber die Resektion der Leber. Sammlung Klinischer Vortrage, Chirurgie, pp 451–530
24. Wendel W (1911) Beitrage zur Chirurgie der Leber. Arch f Klin Chir 95:887–894
25. Tinker MB (1935) Liver resection: case report and advantages of radiocutting. Ann Surg 102:728–741
26. McDill JR (1912) Bloodless surgery of the liver: an experimental study of the possibility of excision of maximum amounts of liver tissue, with the usual instruments at hand in any hospital. Trans Am Surg Assoc 30:106–119
27. McDill JR (1912) Bloodless operations on the liver. Ann Surg 56:333–335
28. Garrè C (1907) On resection of the liver. Surg Gynecol Obstet 5:331–341
29. Miln DC (1964) James Hogarth Pringle, 1863-1941. Br J Surg 51:241–245
30. Pringle JH (1908) Notes on the arrest of hepatic hemorrhage due to trauma. Ann Surg 48:541–546
31. Ponfick E (1890) Ueber leberresection und leberreaction. Verhandl Deutsch Gesellsch Chir 19:28

Chapter 6
The World Wars and Hemorrhage Control

Dangerous abdominal operations such as liver resection could not reasonably advance unless capabilities developed to recognize and address the physiological changes resulting from surgical trauma and loss of blood. This would translate to a better control of the anesthetized patient, more sophisticated monitoring measures, and the ability to quickly resuscitate if blood loss threatened hemodynamic stability.

It seemed that the man-made ravages of the Great War of 1914–1918 (and the ensuing influenza epidemic of 1918) consumed all energy and attention away from the more exotic challenges of visceral surgery. Indeed, the massive numbers of war casualties focused efforts in Germany, France, and England on the immediate resuscitation, repair, and rehabilitation of endless lines of marred and disabled veterans. However, the 1920s saw renewed interest in complex visceral surgery, perhaps with a better understanding of cardiovascular effects of blood loss and fluid resuscitation engendered by war experiences in critically wounded soldiers. Harvard researcher Walter Cannon realized the importance of fluid resuscitation for men in shock by infusion of Ringer's lactate or a concoction of gum acacia developed by British physiologist William Bayliss as plasma expanders.[1] From the efforts of Canadian Bruce Robertson and British-born American naturalized Oswald Robertson blood for transfusion became readily available through preservation and storage and seemed to have a remarkable effect on badly wounded men [2, 3]. Indeed, it seemed a God-send. A century prior blood transfusion pioneer John Henry Leacock spoke in 1817 of the potential miracles of transfusion:

> The consequences of hemorrhage … when danger is imminent and the common means are ineffectual … what reason can be alleged for not having recourse to this last hope, and for not attempting to recruit the exhausted frame, and turn the ebbing tide of life? [4]

And truly, at the turn of the century those early blood transfusions, almost defying nature, seemed agents of miraculous transformation as witnessed by the wife of

---

[1] See Ref. [1], particularly Chap. XXII, "The Treatment of Shock", 174–186

T. S. Helling, D. Azoulay, *Historical Foundations of Liver Surgery*, https://doi.org/10.1007/978-3-030-47095-1_6

the American surgeon George Crile (1864–1943) who was in attendance when her daring husband performed one of the first human-to-human blood transfusions in 1906. She wrote:

> I saw the livid pallor slowly take on a pinkish tinge … So suffused with blood did the patient become that his cheeks, his lips, even his ears, took on a rosy glow … and he began to talk and jest almost like a man intoxicated [5].

At long last, for liver surgeons, the feared consequences of torrential hemorrhage could be countered with infusion of life-giving blood. Modern science now aided the stricken patient, no longer left to their own resilience to surmount surgical assaults. In his presidential address before the American Surgical Association in 1919 Lewis Pilcher commented about the influence of war surgery on civilian practice:

> The careful studies of the subject of shock … such a procedure as blood transfusion … the practical establishment of minute details whereby sepsis was controlled and antisepsis made efficient, and … the surgery of the chest … the abdomen … most important contributions have been made … These in their order and place will occupy our interested attention for years to come [6].

In truth, blood typing, cross matching, and blood preservation revolutionized war surgery—and would revolutionize surgery in general. Now men bled white on the battlefield or in the operating room could undergo resuscitation not only restoring volume but also oxygen-carrying capacity. The mysterious syndrome of traumatic, or wound, shock of World War I gave way to a better understanding of blood depletion with trauma, including surgical trauma, through the brilliant work of Alfred Blalock during the inter-war years. His classic experiments on hind limb trauma in the late 1920s showed without question that the circulatory changes observed after injury were not due to some furtive "toxic factor" but simply to a loss of blood—a totally mechanistic explanation. "Shock … can be produced by hemorrhage alone," he contended. The low blood pressure seen in shock states was no more than loss of volume [7]. The answer? For blood loss give blood.

But monitoring severely traumatized patients, even those undergoing elective, but bloody surgery, demanded some expertise in anesthesia. Indeed, surgery owed anesthesia a debt. Without a profound level of stupor and relaxation, ventures into the abdominal cavity would be almost impossible. The major agents used during and after the First World War—ether, chloroform, and nitrous oxide—were given by dripping the anesthetics onto a cloth covered mask. At the turn of the century the German surgeon Franz Kuhn had begun using metal tubes that he inserted directly through the vocal cords and into the trachea. But it was Sir Ivan Magill (1888–1986) who popularized this method of delivering anesthesia, first used on soldiers with horrific facial injuries from war. Anesthesia could thus be introduced and breathing artificially supported minimizing the untoward effects of insufficient ventilation and airway compromise [8].[2]

---

[2] For an entertaining discussion of the milestones in anesthesia, see Ref. [9].

And until then, level of consciousness and tolerance of the patient were simply monitored by pupillary reflexes and the rate and character of the pulse. Sudden death from these anesthetics was not uncommon, and contributed to the dangers of complex visceral procedures. In 1896, an Italian physician by the name of Scipione Riva-Rocci (1863–1937) had introduced a device he called his sphygmomanometer, a method of measuring blood flow by way of determining arterial pressure. His apparatus he had modified from models developed by predecessors, particularly Karl Vierordt (1818–1884) and Karl von Basch (1837–1905) who featured an instrument "that manometrically measures the force necessary to prevent the progression of the pulse," using a column of mercury [10]. During the war that irrepressible American innovator, George Crile, now serving in France as a member of the American Expeditionary Force, promoted Riva-Rocci's sphygmomanometer as standard fare for use with anesthetized patients, thus linking blood pressure with that dreaded surgical phenomenon of shock. Now, there was another objective measure of hemodynamic stability and tolerance not only of anesthesia but also of the extent of hemorrhage to guide the operating team on proper levels of anesthesia and fluid resuscitation.

George Grey Turner (1877–1951) was small in stature but brimming with enthusiasm and energy. Known to his chums as "GG," the "great little man" was exceedingly admired and loved by those with whom he worked. Many described him as always seeming in a hurry—except in the operating room where he truly thrived, even to the point of introducing a gramophone and a spattering of "Roaring Twenties" jazz into the sanctity of the "Holy of holies" [11].

Turner's curiosity about liver surgery stemmed from the impressionable experience at age 20, of helping one of his mentors, the esteemed George Halliburton, a celebrated surgeon at the Newcastle Infirmary while a medical student at Newcastle-upon-Tyne. He recounted the patient as a 48-year-old woman who had undergone a gastrectomy 18 months prior for cancer. She now presented in June 1897 with an epigastric lump. On exploration the lump proved to be a tumor arising from the edge of the liver just to the left of the gallbladder (the quadrate lobe, or, in today's terminology, segment IVb). Halliburton withdrew "the affected portion of liver from the abdomen, transfixing its base with a couple of knitting needles, and surrounding the pedicle thus formed with an elastic ligature." He then simply cut the tumor away and left the stump extraperitoneal. There was no bleeding. Now on March 1, 1921, he was faced with the same prospect. A 13-year-old boy had presented with a mass on the right side of the abdomen that had caused sudden pain. On performing a right paramedian incision he discovered a large tumor occupying almost one-half of the right lobe of the liver. A frozen section was performed that showed it to be composed of bland liver cells, probably a liver cell adenoma. Turner decided to remove it by a V-shaped incision into the liver. After removal of the gallbladder, he used a "light, bow-shaped stomach clamp with jaws 4 in. long" such as he had used for gastrectomies (similar, it seems, to Kocher's liver clamp). The clamp was placed on the tumor side of his resection and allowed manipulation of the tumor. Then, after the fashion of Kousnetzoff and Pensky, he placed a series of four catgut sutures almost through the liver at the periphery of the tumor, tied the sutures, and cut away the tumor with a knife, maintaining a suitable margin. The small portal pedicles and veins he individually ligated with fine catgut suture. There was some bleeding but nothing alarming. No need for Keen's thermocautery. Finally, he packed gauze over the cut surface and closed. The operation lasted about an hour and a half. Such an undertaking with the potential for disaster and which, as a consequence, deserved the utmost in concentration was totally absorbing. At the end, the completion of this feat was exhilarating. Turner later wrote:

> It is difficult for me to give a word picture of all that happens at an operation of this sort. The conditions are highly unusual, and experience is lacking as to the effect of such a proceeding on the patient, and there is naturally rather an artificial atmosphere of apprehension and excitement … The great problem in dealing with resection of the liver has always been the control of hemorrhage, not only at the time of the operation, but permanently [12]

In this case Turner's attention to detail prevailed. There would be no hemorrhage. The young lad recovered without a hitch and left the hospital 24 days later. He was still doing well 21 months later. The tumor itself was probably an atypical adenoma, although the pathology report claimed a number of mitoses and multinucleated cells.

Turner went on to describe another liver resection he performed on a tumor the size of a closed fist occupying the left lobe and removed it using the same clamping and catgut suturing method as before. But, despite the excitement and satisfaction these two cases provided, Turner put all in perspective. Of the 4935 abdominal operations he had performed, including a number on the liver and biliary system, he had performed only two liver resections, and witnessed a third, all described in this one article.

Yet, prior to World War II, liver resections, even for the most intrepid, were only an occasional dalliance for surgeons. No single practitioner up to that time had much experience beyond a handful of cases. One such surgeon was Martin Tinker from Cornell in New York City. Tinker announce his singular experience with liver surgery at the 1935 meeting of the American Surgical Association in Boston waxing broadly on control of hemorrhage ("[t]his is by far the most important problem in liver resection"), use of autotransfused blood, and techniques of hemostasis, including his "electrocuting and coagulation" (electrocoagulation system)—heretofore used rarely in liver surgery [13]. Tinker apparently preferred the cutting mode as opposed to pure cauterization ("it cuts much faster and I consider it equally efficacious in arresting oozing").[3] He employed his electrosurgery in removing a bleeding hemangioma from the left lobe (lateral section) of a 65-year-old woman, a condition that had proved fatal in other's hands. Blood loss in his patient was apparently modest. Two years later Tinker, now collaborating with his son, Martin, Jr., expounded on liver surgery before the Pan American Medical Association meeting in Havana, Cuba. This presentation was essentially a recap of his American Surgical Association speech. Here the Tinkers emphasized the properties of the liver that favored

---

[3] Electrosurgery was evidently the brainchild of inventor William T. Bovie. He had collaborated with Harvey Cushing to use his new boxy electrical surgery device in removing a brain tumor in 1926. The operation was a smashing success. With Cushing's endorsement, Bovie's electrosurgical unit quickly gained popularity.

resection: the segmental nature of the blood supply and the ability to regenerate. How was resection best achieved? Aside from the proper incision (subcostal) hemorrhage control loomed first and foremost. Inflow occlusion held merit but was a time-limited endeavor—not more than 15 min according to some. Tinker himself had found dramatic drops in blood pressure in experimental animals with portal inflow occlusion, and the distinct concern was for ischemic damage to the intestine [14].

But World War II would see a colossal increase in the use of blood and blood products. The pivotal role of transfusion in cases of traumatic shock was key to the resuscitation of wounded men. In those war years massive traumatic blood loss was matched, in many cases, by the expeditious return of intravenous fluid right on the battlefield. Mutilated men were now arriving within hours of injury for surgeons to begin piecing back together. Internal injuries, previously lethal, were now survivable. The maturation of anesthesiology as a specialty focused on proper administration of anesthetic agents and intraoperative physiologic monitoring, ventilator support, and resuscitative therapy profoundly aided surgeons in opening new frontiers for exploration.[4] Liberal use of banked blood and plasma infusions abrogated some of the feared consequences of massive blood loss inevitable with certain cardiovascular and hepatic operations.

As a result, during World War II, blood usage, either with whole blood or plasma components, was widespread practice. By 1944 the American Red Cross was collecting in excess of 120,000 units to be processed and shipped overseas. Blood transfusion had become standard therapy for traumatic injuries and the pivotal therapy for hemorrhagic shock.[5] At war's end surgeons were eager to apply their military acumen with trauma surgery to the elective conditions of civilian practice. As a result there was renewed interest in the treatment of cancer and the expectation that, with wide extirpation of neoplasms, cure could be effected.

As an outgrowth of World War II, the new specialty of anesthesia would embolden efforts in complex cardiac, vascular, and hepatic procedures. What had been relegated to proficient nurse anesthetists now became a science and medical specialty of its own. From lessons learned in the First World War and through the efforts of pioneers like Harvard-trained Henry Beecher focusing on the cardiopulmonary perturbations of anesthetized patients and their reactions not only to sophisticated anesthetic agents but also the traumatic stress of surgery. Lessons learned during World War II in caring for critically wounded men transferred readily to the civilian scene and formidable elective. Beecher indeed felt that the physiologic response to stress demanded expertise in tending to the anesthetized patient:

> Anesthetists must assume wider burdens than those of clinical anesthesia in its specific sense: The treatment of shock, resuscitation … Anesthetists can be the physiologically—minded guides of therapy in preparation for, during, and immediately following the rigors of surgical intervention [17].

---

[4] For an in-depth review of the emerging role of anesthesia in the European Theater of Operations in World War II, see Ref. [15].

[5] For a detailed summary, see Ref. [16].

The anesthetized subject now benefited greatly from the experience of wartime anesthetists. Almost routine use of endotracheal anesthesia enabled more precise control of hemodynamics and respiratory efforts, a pivotal measure in chest and complex abdominal operations. The presence of a trained and knowledgeable individual at the head of the table enabled surgeons to venture into territory not previously contemplated, knowing that perturbations of cardiovascular stability could be quickly addressed by the anesthesia team [18]. The ability to monitor for subtle changes in body temperature, cardiac rhythm, blood pressure, respiration, and even estimation of blood volume represented substantial progress over that possible just a decade before.[6] The operating room was now more than the surgical theater of the nineteenth century. It had become the physiologic laboratory of twentieth-century medicine. The wails of awake patients, loud boastings and angry shouts of surgeons, and the brutality of speed had been replaced by the rhythmic hum of ventilators, the hushed tones of the operating team, and the merciful obtundation of the anesthetized patient. As Thomas Schlich argued, the "modern" operating room became the new theater for control: surrounded by technologies and antiseptic practices, surgeons now exerted supreme control over disease, or, at least, hoped they could [20]. "Surgical intervention could be represented as the inevitable, scientific solution to disease," so wrote Christopher Lawrence [21]. And none so poignant as surgery of the liver.

The entrepreneurial spirit of surgeons in the decades after World War II was not just due to the wealth of experience that armed conflict engendered. Rapid expansion of the supporting roles of anesthesia and critical surgical care would revolutionize the conduct and daring of surgical intervention. Just as World War I produced remarkable advances in surgical technique, understanding of the physiologic consequences of blood loss and shock, and the rudimentary development of fluid and blood resuscitation of gravely ill patients, the immense bloodshed of World War II propelled resuscitative abilities light years beyond.

References

1. Cannon WB (1923) Traumatic shock. D. Appleton and Company, New York
2. Robertson LB, Watson CG (1918) Further observations on the results of blood transfusions in war surgery with special reference to the results in primary hemorrhage. Ann Surg 67:1–13
3. Robertson OH (1918) Transfusion of preserved red cells. Br J Med 1:691–695
4. Leacock JH (1817) On the transfusion of blood in extreme cases of haemorrhage. Med Chir J Rev 3:276–284
5. Crile G (1947) George Crile: an autobiography. Lippincott, Philadelphia, p 177
6. Pilcher LS (1919) The influence of war surgery upon civil practice. Ann Surg 69:565–574
7. Blalock A (1930) Experimental shock: the cause of the low blood pressure produced by muscle injury. Arch Surg 20:959–996

---

[6] For a detailed explanation of monitoring devices during anesthesia, see Ref. [19].

8. McLachlan G (2008) Sir Ivan Magill KCVO, DSc, MB, BCh, BAO, FRCS, FFARCS (Hon), FFARCSI (Hon), DA, (1888-1986). Ulster Med J 77:146–152

9. Snow SJ (2008) Blessed days of anesthesia. Oxford University Press, Oxford

10. Booth J (1977) A short history of blood pressure measurement. Proc R Soc Med 70:793–799

11. Hedley-Whyte A (1965) George Grey Turner (1877-1951). Br J Surg 52:641–646

12. Turner GG (1923) A case in which an adenoma weighing 2 lb. 3 oz. was successfully removed from the liver: with remarks on the subject of partial hepatectomy. Proc Royal Soc Med 16:43–56

13. Tinker MB (1935) Liver resection: case report and advantages of radiocutting. Ann Surg 102:728–741

14. Tinker MB, Tinker MB Jr (1939) Resection of the liver: conditions favorable for operation; methods; experimental studies. JAMA 112:2006–2008

15. Tovell RM (1964) Anesthesia. In: Coates JB (ed) Activities of the surgical consultants. Office of the Surgeon General, Washington DC, pp 581–621, Medical Department, United States Army

16. Kendrick DB (1964) Blood program in world war II. In: Heaton LD (ed) Medical Department United States Army in World War II. U.S. Government Printing Office, Washington DC, pp 101–137

17. Beecher HK (1947) The specialty of anesthesia and its application in the Harvard University-Massachusetts General Hospital Department. Ann Surg 126:486–499

18. Waisel DB (2001) The role of world war II and the European theater of operations in the development of anesthesiology as a physician specialty in the USA. Anesthesiology 94:907–914

19. Dripps RD (1959) Use of monitoring devices during anesthesia and operation. Perspect Biol Med 2:362–371

20. Schlich T (2007) Surgery, science and modernity: operating rooms and laboratories as spaces of control. Hist Sci 14:231–256

21. Lawrence C (1992) Democratic, divine and heroic: the history and historiography of surgery. In: Lawrence C (ed) Medical theory, surgical practice. Routledge, New York, pp 1–47

Chapter 7
A Worldwide Phenomenon: Liver Surgery in the Far East

Japanese physicians had maintained a close association with German surgery since the Meiji Restoration of 1868, which hoped to reintroduce advances in Western science replacing the previous closed-door attitude of the shogunates. A number of Japanese surgeons had studied under the Teutonic masters Billroth, Vincenz Czerny, Bernhard von Langenbeck, and Ernst von Bergmann and returned to their homeland where a robust Western-style university medical system was developing. The Japanese Surgical Society was founded in 1898 and began annual congresses to showcase Japanese surgical efforts that were far in advance of their mainland Asian colleagues. It was the Japanese delegation to the International Society of Surgery that petitioned for Germany and Austria to be readmitted after the conflagration of World War I [1]. In the interwar period the evolving Nipponese hospital and medical education system was generating admirable clinical results. By the 1930s Japanese surgeon Komei Nakayama reported a remarkably low mortality rate of 16.7% following esophagectomy for cancer [2]. At the same time Hiroshige Shiota had perfected radical methods to eradicate gastric cancer, again with a drastic reduction in operative mortality. While World War II was devastating for Japan's medical system, energetic physician-scholars, with the support of the occupying Allied powers, quickly latched onto American medicine and, from a ruinous health system, began rebuilding the high standards of care they had formerly known.

Ichio Honjo (1913–1987) was born in Tokyo. His medical education and surgical training were all done in Japan, at the Kyoto University School of Medicine. During the war years he was consumed, as were many Japanese physicians, with community service. The devastation and human suffering the United States wrought on his country would overwhelm him and his colleagues until Japan's surrender in 1945. Following Japan's occupation at the end of the war he assumed the position of Chief of Surgery at Kokura Memorial Hospital, in the port city of Fukuoka, on the north shores of Kyoto. He was 32 years old. It was this extraordinary dedication to his craft that would lead Honjo to attempt, and successfully complete, a right hepatic lobectomy (now considered an extended right hepatectomy or right

T. S. Helling, D. Azoulay, *Historical Foundations of Liver Surgery*, https://doi.org/10.1007/978-3-030-47095-1_7

tri-sectionectomy), much as Lortat-Jacob had done, but in 1949, some 2 years earlier. His original description was published in Japanese that same year and not easily accessible or interpretable in the anglophilic West.

In March of 1949 Honjo was asked to see a young man, 22 years old, who had already undergone radical surgery for cancer of the rectum 2 years before. His slender patient had become weaker and had noticed a "tumorous growth" below his right costal margin—Honjo could easily palpate a nodular, hard liver. So, wasting little time, on Monday, March 7, with the aid of colleague Chisato Araki, he embarked on his operation. The incision in this slender young man incorporated a long midline component, a generous extension into the right upper quadrant, and a shorter arm to the left abdomen—a type of cruciate incision. This wide exposure, one could imagine, allowed full access to the patient's liver. Secondly, Honjo then completely mobilized the liver by dividing suspensory ligaments and freeing the posterior "bare" area from the retroperitoneum. Following these maneuvers, Honjo then obtained hilar control of the hepatic artery and portal vein. He planned to take the gallbladder *en bloc* with the right lobe, so he simply ligated and divided the cystic duct, leaving the gallbladder attached. He was not able to encircle the right branch of the hepatic duct, so this was left untouched. Once inflow was controlled Honjo proceeded with the parenchymal resection, using "stout silk sutures" for each of three regions of the liver: the posterior area, containing the major hepatic veins, the *lobus quadratus* (what would later be termed Couinaud segment IV), and "a relatively small portion of liver substance connecting the right lobe with the left." Each of these regions was controlled with one mass ligature of his silk suture. Honjo's major concern throughout was jeopardizing flow to the left liver by impinging on and compromising arterial and portal flow at the hilum. The resected liver, as expected, contained a metastatic adenocarcinoma. Liver function normalized in 1–2 months. There was some postoperative ascites and lower extremity edema, but all resolved in about 2 weeks. While the patient recovered uneventfully from his operation, he developed further recurrences and died less than 18 months later.[1]

Honjo and Araki published this case report in the Japanese journal *Shujutsu* in 1950 [3]. The report was written in Japanese and so escaped the attention of the Western surgical community. It was not until January 1955 that he recapitulated his exploits of 6 years prior in the *Journal of the International College of Surgeons*, acknowledging, with gracious deference and characteristic humility, the achievements of Lortat-Jacob and Robert who, of course, postdated his operation [4]. It is remarkable that in the postwar chaos of Japan two pioneering surgeons were able to complete this daunting task. Even more notable, in December of that same year Honjo performed the first total pancreatectomy. He would devote his career to diseases of the liver, biliary system, and pancreas, receiving numerous awards and accolades until his death in 1987. He would be one of the first true hepato-pancreato-biliary specialists.

---

[1] At autopsy it was found that the middle and left hepatic veins had been preserved, indicating the dissection might have proceeded across Cantlie's line (right hepatectomy) rather than removing the topographic right lobe.

The surgical arts had never developed in ancient or medieval China and, there-fore, Indochina. Despite fanciful legends of miraculous operations (including heart transplants) Chinese surgeons did very little beyond superficial procedures. It is not entirely clear as to why. Anesthesia was not unknown to them, including the magi-cal drug *ma-fei-san* with remarkable sedative properties, likely a mixture of opium and hashish. Certainly, Chinese were familiar with human anatomy. While there were no structured studies of human remains, observations were made on exhumed victims of epidemics and executed criminals. It was permissible, even in ancient times, to dissect the body after death. However, just as with Galen, Chinese anato-mist probably incorporated animal anatomy into human interpretation, assuming one was similar to the other.

Yet, the Chinese were intrigued with the science of splanchnology, the study of internal viscera, and their investigations began over four millennia ago. The liver comprised one of the five parenchymatous organs (heart, spleen, lungs, and kidneys being the other four). The liver, they wrote, had a rancid odor, a sour taste, a brown colon, and was the seat of anger. Yet each of the five organs was to work harmoni-ously and aid in the development of the body. The liver, in that sense, produces the substance to form the heart and control the lungs. The liver, in teleological terms, was to act to mediate the function of the other organs and viscera. In depicting the liver a multilobed structure was diagrammed more suggestive of animal anatomy than human. Even into the nineteenth century Chinese anatomists held to their ancient principles of the gate of life, or source of vitality, as well as rather primitive depiction of anatomic form, even when exposed to Western medicine introduced in China by efforts of missionaries through the trading port of Macao [5].[2] In the eigh-teenth century, the French explorer and missionary to the court of the Manchu emperor Kāngxī Jesuit Dominique Parrenin (1665–1741) wrote that the Chinese were familiar with the flow of blood and lymph but were extremely reluctant to embark on human cadaveric dissection [6]. In fact Parrenin attempted to introduce Western concepts of anatomy, using Thomas Bartholin's *Anatomia Reformata* (1655) as the foundational text, providing explanations and legends in Chinese char-acters and some diagrams in traditional Chinese dress—it was said the entire project took 5 years [7, 8]. Only a few copies, to be known as the "Manchu Anatomy," were allowed by Kāngxī, and these modern depictions of anatomy were never dissemi-nated. Lack of curiosity about human anatomy probably influenced the art of surgery in China. With respect to the state of surgical skills, historian Louis Fu summarized:

> Chinese surgery was of the most barbarous type. No one dared attempt a bloody opera-tion . . . Chinese surgery deteriorated [particularly after popularization of Confucian ide-ology] as it was incompatible with the Chinese religion to sacrifice any part of the body to cure disease [9].

It would be left to Western influence to effect a change. From all reliable sources, surgery was reintroduced by Yale graduate Peter Parker who performed a number of remarkable operations without anesthesia on willing Chinese subjects burdened by

---

[2] A thorough discussion of Chinese anatomy is contained in Ref. [5].

horrible tumors at the Canton Hospital in 1836. "The gratitude and confidence of all classes, from the Imperial Commissioner down to the humblest coolie, were extended to Parker on every side," so wrote historian Harold Balme [10]. William Welch of Johns Hopkins volunteered his knowledge of Chinese surgery in a report before the medical and surgical faculty of Maryland in Baltimore in 1916. The Chinese had a vast *materia medica* and extensive medical writings, but in all that there were very few references to surgery. What was performed was usually at the hands of missionaries who began arriving in the sixteenth century. "They employ their native doctors when anything is the matter with their insides, but for a surgical operation they seek the Western doctor . . .," he found.

In twentieth century Indochina, that exotic frontier sandwiched between the great societies of India and China, surgery, the treatment of conditions and diseases by the hand, was virtually unknown among indigenous populations. Even in traditional Chinese medicine (*Thuốc Bắc*—"northern" medicine), which had heavily influenced Vietnamese practices for centuries, little mention was made of surgery. The arrival of the French and the establishment of a French colonial government allowed the introduction of French educational initiatives to expose the Annamese to "modern" scientific thought and practices.[3] The young gynecologist Du'o'ng-ba-Bành wrote shortly before his untimely death in 1951 that, in Vietnamese medicine, "Surgery is almost nonexistent except for some cutaneous operations or practice of acupuncture." Even in traditional Chinese medicine, the so-called Thuốc Bắc, little mention is made of surgery. Of course there is the legendary Hua Tuo (circa 108–208 AD), regarded as China's first surgeon. Not only a respected surgeon but also a superb herbalist, Hua Tuo used a concoction he called *ma fei san*, a liquid probably containing alcohol and cannabis, as an anesthetic, even employing it to produce unconsciousness in anticipation of abdominal surgery. Much has been lost of the Chinese surgical art through the first millennium until the Middle Ages. Apparently Jesuit fathers, coming to China on missionary work, introduced Western techniques in surgery, mostly, of course, for skin and soft tissue problems.

And so had observed Navy physician Dr. Vialet at the turn of the century. Despite a dazzling knowledge of mineral, vegetable, and animal-based remedies, even some repulsive ones such as compounds of feces from young boys, pigs, cats, and dogs, mixed together that were used for cases of smallpox (before the vaccinations became available), surgery was attempted only rarely. The *indigènes*, who had immense faith in native "wizards," flocked to European doctors for surgical matters. Whether motivated by a fear of harming their patients or by a pecuniary incentive to sell a plethora of medications was uncertain. Nevertheless, to bleed or lance would be a distinctly distasteful undertaking for the Thầy Thuốc. With tongue-in-cheek Vialet added:

For the same reasons should a foreign body come to obstruct the respiratory or digestive tracts, what is the point of trying to find it directly, when one can have so

---

[3] Report of the Book and Journal Club Meeting, March 22, 1916, at which an address was given by Dr. William H. Welch on Medicine in the Orient.

many remedies, all so effective, and one of which, the blood of the comb of a black hen, can bring back life to people who have strangled themselves?

Vialet felt that the root of the problem lay in a childish and fanciful notion of human anatomy. Embedded in ancestral culture was the forbiddance of autopsies so that any knowledge of anatomy would come almost accidentally through terrible mutilations or through extrapolation of animal anatomy. Understanding of physiology, equally important for surgical evolution, was also elemental and, for the most part, irrelevant to any rational treatment. Other than the pulse, which received inordinate amount of attention by local healers, only symptoms obvious to the senses were deemed important. Therapy focused on correction of cold and heat, for the Vietnamese the main causes of disease. The missionary physician Dan Beach Bradley found similar abhorrent practices in midwifery and obstetrics in early nineteenth century Siam. Stubborn deliveries were enhanced by jumping up and down on the gravid uterus, and even with successful parturition, the poor mother had to endure a period of literal roasting before raging fires for a period of 1 month to cleanse mother and infant alike. Needless to say, familiarity with anatomy or inner workings of the pregnant female was largely unknown and awaiting introduction of anatomic plates by patient, diplomatic missionary doctors.

Yet, it was clear that this land, so stunning but so primitive in many respects, sorely needed the introduction of Western medical practices, particularly in the areas of infectious diseases. The increasing demand for public health policies and vaccinations to combat endemic diseases such as smallpox, cholera, and malaria prompted French authorities to implement expanded medical education for Indochinese practitioners. In 1902, *l'École de Médecine de Indochine* (the Indochinese School of Medicine, soon to be called *l'École de Médecine de Hanoi*) was opened to train so-called auxiliary doctors (*médecins auxiliaries*) who would work alongside colonial physicians in more remote areas of the protectorates (Tonkin, Annam, Cambodia, Laos, and Cochinchina). By the 1920s native Indochinese (mostly Vietnamese) were able to obtain a full-fledged medical degree with the same standing as their French faculty. Nevertheless, specialty training, particularly in surgery, lagged behind.[4]

Here is where the story of Tôn Thất Tùng (1912–1982) begins (Figs. 7.1 and 7.2). This young Vietnamese was a mandarin's son, from the imperial city of Hue on the banks of the Perfume River. Following his secondary education, Tùng ventured off to Hà Nội in the northern French protectorate of Tonkin and was selected for medical studies at *l'Ecole de Médecine de Hanoi*.[5] Tùng learned well at the hands of his French instructors. In fact, he would become the first Indochinese to be selected for training in surgery. Tùng had tremendous energy and enthusiasm. Not wasting any opportunities to learn, he spent his spare time assisting in autopsies. It

---

[4] For elaboration on medical education in Indochina, see Ref. [11].

[5] Tonkin would eventually fold into "North Vietnam" after the defeat of the French at Điện Biên Phủ in 1954 and until the unification of all of Vietnam following the American exodus and conquest of "South" Vietnam in 1975.

Fig. 7.1 Vietnamese
surgeon Professor Ton That
Tung (1912–1982). Photo
courtesy of CTV/CVN

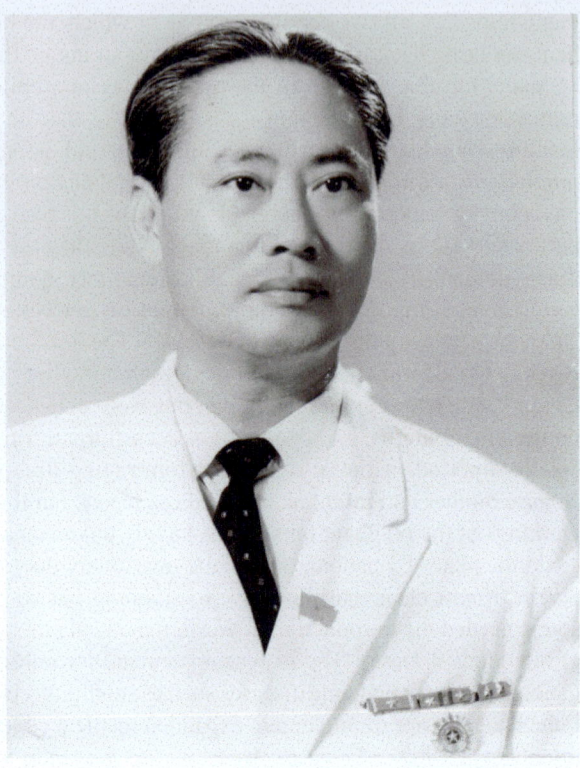

Fig. 7.2 Ton That Tung
lecturing medical students
during the war years. Photo
courtesy of CTV/CVN

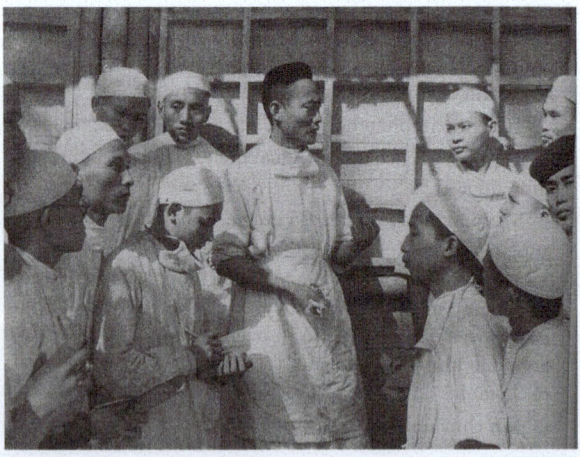

was there that he developed a keen interest in the liver because of the ubiquitous
presence of the roundworm, which he could track into the biliary ducts on autopsy
specimens. This led, of course, to a curiosity of the entire intrahepatic architecture.
By using casting methods and dissection of over 200 human livers, Tùng

demonstrated that blood flow in the liver, the interdigitating relationships of portal and hepatic veins, was regional, not haphazard, and therefore lent itself to regional (segmental) anatomic demarcation. For the surgeon this implied the ability to remove portions of the liver without compromising neighboring regions.[6] That finding was not lost on Tùng who was anxious to embark on liver surgery. Tùng approached his chief mentor at the time, Jacques Meyer-May with his idea of segmental liver resection. "I proposed to him my technique of hepatic resection which he warmly welcomed but not without some apprehension," Tùng would later relate in his memoirs [12].[7]

On their own, without much liver experience or the benefit of European masters, he and Meyer-May performed two left hepatic "lobectomies"—what would today be called left lateral sectionectomies—in 1938 and 1939, both for hepatocellular carcinoma.[8] Their first patient harbored a large tumor of the topographical left lobe, thought at first to be a metastasis from gastric cancer but, after resection, proved to be a primary hepatocellular carcinoma. The operation was successful. "I crushed the hepatic tissue with pincers, leading the way for Professor Meyer May to expose and clamp the vessels," Tùng recalled in his autobiography [12].[9] The patient survived the operation and lived for 5 months, dying of recurrent disease. Proud of their accomplishments, the two pioneers submitted a paper to the *Académie Nationale de Chirurgie* in Paris. It was published in the Mémoires de l'Académie de Chirurgie for November 22, 1939. In his discussion of the paper Professor Paul Funk-Brentano of the *Académie* gave a scathing reply, chastising both surgeons for operating on a hopeless cancer and not affording the patient the benefit of the most modern techniques (employing thermocautery). His implication was that an impoverished country like Tonkin had no business doing surgery of this magnitude. Funk-Brentano would comment:

> Except very rare exception (targeting cases of malignant trabecular adenoma), it is therefore experimental surgery which provides, to use the expression of the authors of the observation reported today, the opportunity to perform on the living an operation which seems so simple in the cadaver

"I will conclude," he went on to say, "it is a very irrational operation given the extreme uncertainty of the diagnosis of primary liver cancer."[10]

Tùng was crushed. Such a rebuke from the pillars of academia were devastating. And, to add injury to insult, their second patient died on the operating table, a victim

---

[6] It is doubtful that, at the time, Tùng was familiar with the works of either Rex or Cantlie, even though they are later mentioned in his publications.

[7] Excerpts also found in Ref. [13].

[8] Actually, Meyer-May was no stranger to liver resection. He and fellow French surgeon Pierre Huard had previously reported a left lobectomy for a liver abscess in 1936 [14].

[9] Tùng, *Reminiscences*, p 22.

[10] Report by P. Funk-Brentano on [15].

of some type of vascular torsion producing sudden vascular collapse. This dampened enthusiasm for the young Vietnamese. It was not until the liberation of Hanoi from the French in 1954 that Tôn Thất Tùng would return to his first passion, liver surgery.

But he then indulged with a vengeance. By 1962, Tùng had performed 56 liver resections, including six topographical right lobectomies (extended right hepatectomies). His overall mortality was, for the times, a respectable 17%, although two of his six right lobectomies died [16].

What singled Tôn Thất Tùng out, however, was his solid knowledge of anatomy and his ability to wed it to his surgical technique. Tùng understood the segmental nature of liver substance and used it to guide his operative approach. Such wisdom produced almost bloodless surgery. Moreover, at the *Phủ Doãn* Hospital in Hà Nội he used Pringle's maneuver of portal clamping and employed controlled hypotension and hypothermia, placing the patient in a bath tub filled with ice and dropping the body temperature to 30 °C. And Tùng became the master of what was later called *digitoclasie* (finger-fracture), pressing liver tissue between thumb and forefinger, until only vessels remained. Not one to waste time, Tùng preferred the intraparenchymal control of portal pedicles rather than hilar ligation. This technique also favored segmental resections as a means to preserve liver tissue and minimize the resected portion (he performed a total of 42 in his series of 56 resections).[11] He was of such renown in France that he toured the liver centers of Paris, the clinics of Jacques Hepp, Henri Bismuth, and even Lortat-Jacob giving talks and demonstrations [12].[12]

But Tôn Thất Tùng was a victim of the isolationism that was thrust on the new nation of Vietnam due to her struggles for independence first with the French and later the Americans. Scientific progress under Communist rule was sequestered behind the Iron Curtain and either went unnoticed or fell under the skepticism of Western scientists. As a result, there was little recognition of his achievements. He managed only one publication in the English language literature, an article in *The Lancet*, published in January 1963, in which Tùng reiterated his principles of successful liver resection: use of hypothermia, portal clamping in anticipation of resection, and separation of parenchyma using *digitoclasie* and ligature [18]. Still, Western medicine was not convinced.[13] Yet, undaunted, by 1977 Tùng had performed almost 500 liver resections, over two-thirds being segmental resections. He was one of the first surgeons to focus primarily on the liver, pausing in his career only to serve his countrymen in time of war and then to assiduously build the infrastructure of medical science in his new country. His interest in liver surgery, though, would dominate his career, and he continued to advocate the importance of a thorough understanding of anatomy for proper surgical technique.

---

[11] See Ref. [17]; it is not clear where Tùng learned *digitoclasie*. Other Asian surgeons employed it (Lin in Taiwan). It may be that his French colleagues were adept at it and taught him.

[12] Tùng, *Reminiscences*, p 64–65.

[13] Notable exceptions were the French who considered Tùng a remarkable and extremely gifted surgeon.

On the island of Formosa at the turn of the twentieth century, diseases of the liver were predominately infectious in nature, the most feared of which were tropical: amebic abscesses, often preceded, of course, by amebic dysentery. The feared result was rupture of the abscess into the peritoneal cavity, a consequence that was invariably fatal. The only justifiable treatment, it was said, "is surgical interference at the earliest possible moment, with marsupialization of the abscess wall to the parietes [parietal peritoneal surfaces]." Neoplasms were infrequently encountered. While cirrhosis was not uncommon and rarely associated with alcohol intake, no mention was made of an association with cancer. Three cases only of primary cancer of the liver were recorded (almost certainly more were present but undetectable), none of which were resected [19].

Following arrival of missionaries in mid-nineteenth century, it became apparent that only wounds and skeletal trauma were treated in a quasi-surgical nature, although there continued to be heavy reliance on herbal medicine. Medical missionary Dr. James Maxwell arrived in 1865 and introduced Western medicine to the indigenous population, establishing clinics throughout the countryside and impacting health care for infectious diseases.[14] In 1879, work began on a new, Western-style hospital in Tainan that would not be completed until after the Japanese occupation of 1896. With the end of the First Sino-Japanese War in 1895, the Qing Dynasty ceded to Japan the island of Formosa (Treaty of Shimonoseki). The earliest hospital, called *Sin-lâu* Hospital in Tainan provided the first formal operating room on the island. Although Presbyterian missionaries attempted to teach some medicine, a medical school was not established until 1899 by the Japanese, formalizing instruction in European medicine. By 1900 Scottish missionary George Mackay observed "In matters of surgery the natives acknowledge the superiority of foreign practitioners, but in dealing with internal diseases preeminence is claimed for their own doctors." "I have no more faith in the prescriptions of the native doctors than I have in those of priests or sorcerers" [21]. Arrival of Japanese colonist was instrumental in setting up medical colleges for the training of indigenous doctors, supervised by Japanese and missionary faculty. Perhaps the most influential role the Japanese played as Formosa's colonists was the introduction of more modern medical practices. Nevertheless, until 1940 most Taiwanese practitioners were graduates of vocational schools or medical colleges of clinical practice. Less than 5% would attain a university degree. The Japanese system very much resembled the French medical training for indigenous Indochinese [22].

Taiwanese Professor Tien-Yu Lin (1913–1995) had always believed that heaven determined the success of a man's actions. He was indeed a spiritualist. And the Chinese character "Yu" in Tien-*Yu* Lin was meant to indicate "spirit" rather than the more common interpretation "person." Professor Lin was much more than that, not just another "person." His true greatness would emanate from his infectious spirit. He was born in 1913 in Taipei, Taiwan. His family was poor and as a child he was more interested in ducks than studies. That soon changed. A friend's house contained many books, and Lin became a voracious reader. He graduated from Taipei

---

[14] For further discussion of the Presbyterian medical missions see [20].

Normal College and was accepted into Taihoku Medical College in 1936.[15] It was there that his fascination with anatomy and surgery blossomed. After graduation he stayed on at the Taihoku Imperial University Hospital as an unsalaried assistant to Professor Zawada who served as the young student's mentor for several years. Following his surgical training and the liberation of Taiwan from the Japanese in 1945, Dr. Lin was appointed to the faculty of the newly renamed National Taiwan University Hospital. By 1952 he had attained the rank of Professor, and by 1954 he was head of the Department of Surgery. Professor Lin was a true visceral surgeon, focusing on the entire gastrointestinal tract. His first clinical adventure, after a period of study in America, was in thoracic surgery, pioneering the use of general anesthesia for thoracotomy and esophageal resections for carcinoma. Because of the high incidence of primary liver cancer in Taiwan, Lin developed a deepening interest in the causes and treatment. By 1958 Lin and his team had performed four left hepatic lobectomies for cancer. All patients survived. Three of those patients were presented in the *Journal of the Formosan Medical Association* in 1958 [24]. Although his reputation preceded him, Lin had a commanding presence. He was a tall imposing figure—intimidating to those who did not know him. Yet he was soft-spoken, kind, considerate of those around him. In the operating room all was quiet. Lin worked carefully, slowly, meticulously. Absolute control of his environment was key for operations as complex and dangerous as liver surgery.

This demeanor eventually paid dividends. On August 4, 1958, a 36-year-old man was found to have a lump in the right epigastrium. Lacking any diagnostic imaging Lin and his team felt that the tumor occupied the right liver. Their endoscopy had shown that the duodenum was pressed medially, indicating a right-sided lesion. On August 10 Lin performed the first total right lobe resection in Taiwan. His technique involved a thoraco-abdominal incision, using a transverse opening and extending it across the eighth interspace into the chest when he found the tumor was resectable. The cystic duct and artery were transected, the gallbladder left attached to the right lobe. He then embarked on a splitting of the liver using what he termed "finger-fracture." The thumb and index finger were inserted directly into liver tissue and the tissue then "smashed to pieces." When any resistant structure was encountered it was clamped, ligated, and divided. His practice was to ligate and divide portal vein, hepatic artery, and hepatic duct within the liver substance, similar to the method of Tung.[16] Blood replacement during the procedure totaled 2500 mL. The specimen itself weighed 1 kg and measured 14 by 12 by 9 cm. It was, in fact, a hepatocellular carcinoma. The patient dutifully recovered and was alive and well for over 1 year. He eventually died of pulmonary metastases 19 months later.

One month later he completed the second right liver resection on a 6-month-old baby girl. Again, a palpable mass was felt in the upper abdomen and a barium

---

[15] Taihoku Medical College was established in 1922 under the auspices of the Japanese. In 1936, Taihoku (Taipei) Imperial University was founded and a school of medicine created. After liberation from the Japanese in 1945 the name was changed to College of Medicine, National Taiwan University [23].

[16] While not acknowledging Tung (or vice-versa), Lin's technique is eerily similar to that described by Tung almost contemporaneously.

Fig. 7.3 The Lin liver clamp applied (arrow shows ischemic, clamped liver). Adapted from Lin TY

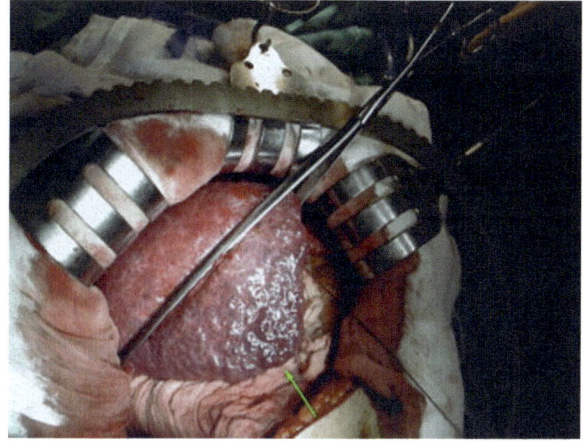

contrast study showed displacement of the stomach to the left, indicating a right-sided tumor. Again, the finger-fracture method was used. The resected "liver cell carcinoma" (probably hepatoblastoma) weighed 370 g and measured 12 by 11.5 by 7 cm. The small child had an uneventful postoperative course.[17]

Professor Lin was probably best remembered in the Western world for his "Lin" liver clamp (Fig. 7.3). He invented the clamp because, as he observed, blood loss during liver surgery could be "considerable" and during "this particular period [finger-fracture] a sense of insecurity often plagues the surgeon"—and indeed, according to his descriptions, the operations liberated blood freely. The clamp was to be placed across the remnant liver prior to transection, the inferior blade being passed on top of the retrohepatic inferior vena cava along the avascular plane and ideally incorporating the respective hepatic veins. The finger-fracture technique was then used to separate liver tissue and effect the resection. The procedure as reported in two patients dramatically reduced blood loss [26].

Despite his keen interest in liver cancer and his pioneering efforts in liver resection he continued to be the consummate general surgeon; Lin began performing cardiac surgery at Taihoku Hospital in 1956 and accomplished the first open-heart operation in 1964 for a ruptured aneurysm of the sinus of Valsalva. He also encouraged development of kidney transplantation and stayed involved in endocrine and gastrointestinal surgery. During his lifetime, though, he would perform over 700 liver resections.[18] Outside of his home country of Taiwan Lin would always be associated with his contributions to liver surgery. Yet, like many of his contemporaries, with such diversified interests he would be a "man for all seasons."

---

[17] Both cases described in Ref. [25].

[18] Anecdotal stories about Professor Lin are contained in a touching tribute to him on the occasion of his 80th birthday in 1993 *The Silent Giant: A Tribute to Professor Tien-Yu Lin on the Occasion of his Eightieth Birthday* [translated by Christopher MacDonald] (Taipei: Chinfon Global Corp, 1992).

References

1. Liebermann-Meffert D, White H (2001) A century of international Progress and tradition in surgery. Kaden, Heidelberg, p 220
2. Nakayama K (1952) Surgery of the esophagus. Nippon Rinsho Geka Gakkai Zasshi 53:1–43
3. Honjo IA, Araki C (1950) 肝臓右葉(亜)全切除に就て [Total resection of the right lobe of the liver]. Shujutsu 4:345–349; [in Japanese]
4. Honjo I (1955) Total resection of the right lobe of the liver: report of a successful case. J Int Coll Surg 23:23–28
5. Hsieh ET (1920) A review of ancient Chinese anatomy. Anat Rec 20:97–124
6. Parrenin RP (1770) Lettres Contenant Diverses Questions sur la Chine, 1st edn. Royal Printing House, Paris, p 17
7. Young TK-H (1974) French Jesuits and the "Manchu anatomy"—how China missed the Vesalian revolution. CMA J 111:565–568
8. Huard P (1953) La Diffusion de l'Anatomie Europeenne dans Quelques Secteurs de l'Asie. Arch Int Hist Sci 32:266–278
9. Fu L (2009) Surgical history of ancient China, part 1. ANZ J Surg 79:879–885
10. Balme H (1921) China and modern medicine. United Council for Missionary Education, London, pp 42–44
11. Monnais L, Thompson CM, Wahlbert A (eds) (2012) Southern medicine for southern people. Cambridge Scholars Publishing, Newcastle upon Tyne
12. Tùng TT (1980) Reminiscences of a Vietnamese surgeon. Foreign Languages Publishing House, Hanoi
13. Tung TT (1993) Đường Vào Khoa Học Của Tôi [My Road to Science]. Youth Publishing House, Hanoi, p 20
14. Huard P, Meyer-May J (1936) Les Abces du Foie. Masson et Cie, Paris
15. Meyer-May J, Tung TT (1939) Résection Anatomique du Lobe Gauche du Foie pour Cancer. Guérison Opératoire et Survie de Cinq Mois. Mem Acad Chir 65:1208–1216
16. Tung TT (1939) La Vascularisation Veineuse du Foie et ses Applications aux Resections et Lobectomies Hepatique. Taupin & Cie, Hanoi
17. Tung TT (1962) Chirurgie D'exerese du Foie. Masson & Cie, Hanoi
18. Tung TT (1963) A new technique for operating on the liver. Lancet 1:192–193
19. Jefferys WH, Maxwell JL (1910) The diseases of China including Formosa and Korea. John Bale Sons & Danielsson, London, pp 240–246; 324–326
20. Johnston J (1897) China and Formosa: the story of the mission of the Presbyterian church of England. Fleming H. Revell Co., New York, pp 301–331
21. Mackay GL (1900) From far Formosa: the island, its people and missions. Oliphant, Anderson & Ferrier, Edinburgh, p 310, 313
22. Shiyung Liu M (2017) Transforming medical paradigms in 1950s Taiwan. East Asia Tech Soc 11:477–497
23. Ha H, Gao T (2002) Centenary history of the College of Medicine, National Taiwan University. Zhonghua Yi Shi Za Zhi 32:163–169, (in Chinese, Chinese Journal of Medical History)
24. Lin T-Y, Hsu K-Y, Hsich C-M, Chen C-S (1958) Study on lobectomy of the liver: a new technical suggestion on hemihepatectomy and reports of 3 cases of primary hepatoma treated with total left lobectomy of the liver. J Formosan MA 57:742–761
25. Lin T-Y, Chen K-M, Liu TK (1960) Total right hepatic lobectomy for primary hepatoma. Surgery 48:1048–1060
26. Lin T-Y (1973) Results in 107 hepatic lobectomies with a preliminary report on the use of a clamp to reduce blood loss. Ann Surg 177:413–421

Chapter 8
Beginning the Modern Era

As it turns out, the Japanese pioneering surgeon Ichio Honjo may have been the second surgeon to successfully resect the topographic right liver lobe but his feat was followed quickly by Dr. Owen Wangensteen (1898–1981) (so Lortat-Jacob may have been the *fourth* to resect the right lobe). Owen Wangensteen, the brilliant Minnesotan, who, at the age of 32 was appointed surgeon-in-chief of the University of Minnesota Hospitals, reported an operation on a 45-year-old man who was previously treated for cancer of the stomach with a subtotal gastrectomy 1 year prior. He was operated again on November 30, 1949, by the Minnesota team and found to have a right lobe of his liver almost totally replaced by tumor. "The entire right lobe" was then removed. Bleeding was limited by the application of occlusive clamps, so-called "Blalock clamps" to the hepatic artery, superior mesenteric artery, and portal vein.[1] The hepatic veins were ligated as they were encountered, working through the liver substance. Bleeding was not mentioned and was apparently minimal. The specimen weighed 872 g and consisted almost entirely of metastatic adenocarcinoma. In fact, a second nodule in the left lobe was also enucleated. The patient's recovery was complicated by a successfully drained subphrenic abscess, but he eventually died on June 30, 1950, about 7 months later, apparently of recurrent disease [1].

Following Lortat-Jacob's widely publicized liver resection there seemed to be an explosion of reports of successful hepatic resections. One notable example was the surgery of George Pack, head of the Gastric Service at Memorial Cancer Center in New York City, and Harvey Baker, one of his fellows, who performed a right hepatic lobectomy in December 1952 for a giant tumor later proved to be a plasma cell granuloma. George Pack was a true surgical oncologist, first training in pathology, then the infant field of radiation therapy, and finally surgery. He was appointed

---

[1] The "Blalock" vascular clamp was designed by Alfred Blalock's talented assistant, Vivien Thomas and a young upstart, William Longmire, working with a local surgical supply house. The clamp was originally designed as a screw-type device with cushioned teeth to gently occlude the pulmonary artery.

T. S. Helling, D. Azoulay, *Historical Foundations of Liver Surgery*,
https://doi.org/10.1007/978-3-030-47095-1_8

Chief of the Gastric Service at Memorial Hospital in New York but his work (and writings) extended to liver, melanomas, sarcomas, rectal cancers, and breast cancer [2]. Of course, the liver surgery he reported was a monumental undertaking for the time. The entire affair was done through a generous thoracic and abdominal incision, affording wide exposure to the right portion of the liver. Like many others, Pack chose to control hepatic inflow with, first, ligation of the right hepatic artery, right hepatic duct, and right branch of the portal vein at the hilum of the liver. He then rotated the liver out of the abdomen by dividing lateral and superior attachments and then, peering underneath, ligated minor hepatic veins (perhaps even the main right hepatic vein). His parenchymal dissection included the quadrate lobe indicating that this was a true topographic right lobectomy. The operation was bloody. Pack commented "the bleeding encountered on severing the right from the left lobe of the liver … was profuse." Surely, without the new luxury of blood transfusion the patient would not have survived. Four thousand milliliters of whole blood was given during the surgery. Surprisingly, there was prompt function of the remaining liver due to, in Pack's words, "compensatory hypertrophy" of the contralateral liver, as the right side was almost totally replaced with neoplasm [3].[2]

Indeed, by the late 1950s for adventurous surgeons worldwide the liver had become fair game. While it remains a mystery how many surgeons performed these daunting operations (or their outcomes), one can only focus on those whose experience was more positive and deserving of comment in publications and presentations.[3] In doing so, a rough mosaic begins to appear of subtle philosophies, techniques, tools, and proficiencies that, in the aggregate, moved the art forward. One such contributor was the Italian surgeon Vittorio Pettinari (1901–1967). Under the fascist regime of Benito Mussolini Pettinari had studied extensively in France and Milan in visceral surgery and become a primary surgeon at the Ospedale di Milano-Niguarda in 1938. He had reported his first case of liver resection in 1940—a left lobectomy—during which he introduced his *Elektromessers* (electric knife), probably a form of electrocautery, to divide liver substance.

By 1959 Pettinari was convinced that surgery of the liver should be standard treatment for hepatic tumors. "Now that certain erroneous biological conceptions have been corrected, radical surgery of the liver is more or less in line with the most up-to-date approaches to internal surgery," he penned. As director of the *Istituti di Patologia e Clinica Chirurgica* in Padua, he had already amassed 41 cases of liver resection, including three primary and seven "secondary" malignant tumors and six cases of tumors of the gallbladder or bile ducts. His success was more or less in line with others. Five of his patients had died, among them two with cirrhosis [6].

Like his contemporaries, Pettinari characterized his resections as major or minor, or, in Pettinari's words "typical" and "atypical." Atypical resections were less

---

[2] Pack was fascinated with the phenomenon of hepatic regeneration, studying the process in his laboratory in rats. For further details see [4, 5].

[3] It is likely that many unreported hepatic operations ended in disaster. For the ill-prepared surgeon massive bleeding often resulted in poor inflow control and failure to appreciate the complex internal anatomy of the liver. Surgeons are notorious (as are journal editors) for underreporting such misadventures.

agreeable. Pettinari's "segmentectomy," as he called it, was a bloody, difficult affair and one to be discouraged. "On the right side this [segmentectomy] is of little practical interest," he later remarked, "since the segmental hila lie deep in the liver and the superficial boundaries cannot be marked out precisely" [7]. "There does not seem … to be much likelihood of its being widely used in the future," he wrote in 1962. His major objection? The seemingly random intrahepatic branchings gave no clear dissection plane and opened up constant opportunities for blood loss.

On the other hand, typical resections, such as right and left hepatectomies, were more anatomically pleasing and reasonable, albeit undertaken with a certain judiciousness. "[T]hose which require section of the parenchyma along the longitudinal scissurae are practicable and fully justified."

> Left lobectomy which is a fairly easy operation incurring little risk in expert hands and is very well tolerated has many indications. … Right lobectomy … is a serious operation which involves hepatic destruction of such an extent as to order on the limits of tolerability; the slightest technical error … abnormalities of vasculature, conditions tending further to reduce the surface and function of the parenchyma are factors liable to cause a fatal result.[4]

Woe to the ill-prepared surgeon, then. How quickly blunders occurred and how steep the penalty for such miscalculations. Liver surgery demanded the utmost in training, skill, patience, vigilance, and readiness.

More mosaics. An obscure Georgia physician named Julian Quattlebaum would rise to prominence as a pioneer in hepatic surgery. Son of a Georgia physician Julian had no formal surgical training. He finished medical school at the Medical College of Georgia in 1921 and settled in Savannah to open a surgical practice. Through visits at major medical centers, his favorite being the Mayo Clinic in Rochester, Minnesota (because of its proximity to baseball games in Chicago and the Indianapolis 500), Quattlebaum quickly picked up the anatomic knowledge and manual skills requisite for surgery. Despite his unorthodox training he earned the respect of colleagues across the country, becoming a Fellow of the American College of Surgeons and a member of the prestigious Southern Surgical Association [9]. Whether he was aware of the exploits of fellow countryman Wangensteen or even the Frenchman Lortat-Jacob is uncertain,[5] but at the Southern Surgical Association meeting in Hollywood, Florida, on December 10, 1952, Dr. Quattlebaum reported on three patients on whom he had performed "massive resection[s] of the liver." Each patient had a right hepatic lobectomy, one coupled with resection of the head of the pancreas.[6] Each patient survived the surgery. For his exposure, Quattlebaum preferred a wide transverse abdominal incision with an extension upward across the costal cartilage. Like others, he favored hilar ligation of portal

---

[4]All quotes from [8].

[5]Lortat-Jacob published his now famous report in *Presse Medicale* on April 16, 1952, and in French. It is doubtful Quattlebaum knew of this at the time of his presentation to the Southern Surgical Association in December that same year.

[6]Apparently this was a pancreatic neuroendocrine tumor with an isolated hepatic metastasis. It is remarkable that Quattlebaum, conducting a community practice in Savannah, was able to complete this feat at the unimpressive Oglethorpe Sanitarium, a three-story brick structure built in 1908 in Savannah (since razed) with modest operative capabilities.

vein, hepatic artery, and hepatic duct, and divided liver parenchyma using the handle of a knife. His plane of transection was near the falciform ligament, identifying each of these as a topographic right lobectomy.[7] The report was subsequently published in *Annals of Surgery* in June 1953. On the cover of one of the reprints of his publication Dr. Quattlebaum scribbled "this article puts me with big leagues." And indeed it did. Julian Quattlebaum focused his practice on liver and biliary surgery, presenting his work twice more at the Southern Surgical Association and becoming internationally recognized for his interest in liver disease. His son, Julian Jr., followed in his father's footsteps. The younger Julian also graduated from the Medical College of Georgia (1951) but then received his surgery training at the Johns Hopkins Hospital. He returned to Savannah to practice with his father and remained there his entire career. Together, father and son published their technique for liver resection in 1959 (also read before the Southern Surgical Association in 1958), describing five important steps in approaching this daunting operation: adequate exposure; complete mobilization; hilar control of vessels; blunt division of liver substance; and ligation of intrahepatic vessels with fine silk or cotton—enduring principles in liver surgery [10].

With the remarkable advances in surgical therapy engendered by World War II came a renewed interest in the aggressive surgical treatment of cancer, a disease historically perplexing and relentless in its progression. For many physicians extirpation was the rational treatment. In fact, for surgeons, more was better. Radical removal of cancerous tumors with generous margins of healthy tissue would, so it was thought, eliminate those subtle, microscopic nests of cells beyond the main tumor and effect a cure. And the liver was an untapped reservoir of neoplasms, both primary and metastatic—an organ that was the frequent haven for cancer's inexorable march across the human landscape.

One early advocate of resection of even metastatic tumors was a square-jawed, ruggedly handsome Ohioan by the name of Richard Cattell (1900–1964). A Quaker and grandson of a staunch abolitionist, Cattell was born in Martins Ferry, on the banks of the Ohio River. Imbued with Quaker qualities of tolerance, equality, and pacifism, Cattell was drawn to medicine at an early age. A likely mentor was his uncle Richard Brenneman, a surgeon. At age 17 Cattell enlisted in the Army Medical Corps and spent a year at Evacuation Hospital No. 2 in France with the American Expeditionary Forces. Following his return it was Mount Union College (Phi Beta Kappa), Harvard Medical School (Alpha Omega Alpha) and on to internship at New England Deaconess. Doctor Cattell completed his surgical residency at Saint Luke's Hospital in Manhattan in 1927 (a two-year stent) and took a position at the Lahey Clinic outside Boston, from which he never left. His surgical acumen and manual skills quickly brought him notoriety, referred to as "Rapid Richard" by residents for the speed at which operations were completed. Young surgeons had a "profound desire to emulate him," a surgical fellow commented in 1945. And there was a

---

[7] It is likely that Quattlebaum's first case was only a few weeks apart from Lortat-Jacob's well publicized affair in Paris.

relentless curiosity about visceral disorders that led Cattell to focus on pancreatic, biliary, and colonic disorders. In fact, his performance of the Miles procedure (staged abdomino-perineal resection for rectal cancer) was so efficient that the whole 75 min affair was called Cattell's "hour of charm" [11]. It was during one of those cases in July 1939 that Cattell stumbled onto an isolated liver metastasis, over three inches in diameter, in the anatomic right lobe (now known as Segment IVb of the left liver) in a 70-year-old woodsman. Finding no other evidence of metastatic spread, Cattell unabashedly proceeded with a large wedge-type resection. Bleeding in this cavernous divot was controlled with "slow, coagulating current" and separate ligatures. Both faces were brought together with individual catgut sutures, and Cattell continued with the first stage of his Miles operation (division of the sigmoid colon and proximal colostomy).[8] His liver tumor, of course, proved to be an adenocarcinoma of rectal origin. One month later the perineal part of his staged operation was successfully performed. Twelve months after that his surgeon reported the patient was in "excellent condition" [13].

Richard Cattell did not achieve fame by his pioneering work in metastatic liver disease. His *forte* remained surgery of the pancreas and bile ducts, even operating on Sir Anthony Eden, the British Foreign Secretary under Winston Churchill in 1953 following a bile duct injury from his cholecystectomy. Supremely confident in the operating room, Cattell filled the air not with pomposity but with a serene calm that was infectious. "He seemed to have things so in hand that emotional upset simply would serve no purpose," a fellow testified. Certainly a tranquil demeanor and meticulous attention to bleeding vessels coupled with gentle, patient forbearance were ideal traits for hepatobiliary surgeons, when expeditious identification of vessels and control of hemorrhage is key to success (and, in some cases, survival).

And there were other early surgical oncologists. Alexander Brunschwig (1901–1969) was one of the first, his intentions to eradicate cancer by wide, sweeping resections. Those were the days when scientists thought of cancer's evolution as a logical, stepwise process from primary site to regional lymph nodes and on to distant metastatic spread. This was the basis for radical, expansive resections. There was really nothing else to offer. In the 1940s and 1950s chemotherapy was in its infancy, of no practical value for solid tumors. Surgery, and only surgery, held hope for cure.

Alexander Brunschwig was born in El Paso, Texas, the son of immigrant parents from Alsace-Lorraine. Driven by an outstanding intellect (and an allergy to horses) he left Texas and completed undergraduate and graduate (Masters) studies at the University of Chicago. His enormous energy was not satiated, however, and Brunschwig soon enrolled in Rush Medical College for his medical education. An internship at Boston City Hospital in pathology fueled his interest in oncology. After further surgical training at the University of Chicago he stayed on as a member of the faculty there. Brunschwig attacked solid visceral tumors with a vengeance

---

[8] William Ernest Miles (1869–1947) was an English surgeon who perfected a two-stage operation for carcinoma of the rectum and published his experience in 1908. The second stage consisted of the perineal excision of the rectum and mesorectum. See Ref. [12].

in a variety of uncompromising abdominal operations: abdomino-perineal resections for rectal cancer, eviscerating pelvic exenterations, radical gastrectomy for stomach cancer, and converting the pancreaticoduodenectomy of Whipple, Barclay, and Mullins to a one-stage operation in 1937. Even widespread metastatic disease did not dissuade him, convinced that removal of visible tumor would extend life. In 1945, Brunschwig reported 100 patients who had his style of aggressive treatment for intra-abdominal cancer, including a number of partial liver resections.[9] The results were dismal. Over one-third of his cases died postoperatively, and only 12 percent surviving long term [14]. Nevertheless, Brunschwig's "ultra-radical" surgery caught the attention of clinicians at New York's Memorial Hospital in 1947 where he moved to become Chief of Gynecology. Despite a focus on gynecological cancers, his interest remained eclectic—including surgery on the liver. In 1953, Brunschwig published a review of 33 patients who had undergone liver resection (since 1947). There were four operative deaths, all in patients who had resection of the right lobe, two of which may have had some type of alcohol-induced chronic liver disease [15]. Two years later Brunschwig updated his experiences with major liver resections, 12 left lobectomies and 10 right lobectomies. Only one of his left-sided resections died but he continued to struggle with right lobectomies. Now half had died in the perioperative period of "shock" (an additional patient died after 1 month of carcinomatosis). Some of these particular patients, he scribed, "were very desperate cases, indeed." His assessment of the high mortality of right-sided liver surgery? "Little need be added by way of discussion of right hepatic lobectomies. It is an operation that is established and has its proper indications," Brunschwig concluded. In cases of cancer, any risk was worth the effort, he seemed to think [16].

For a few surgeons in those postwar days the liver and bile ducts became a primary interest. In the United States the athletic-looking William Longmire Jr. (1913–2003), son of an Oklahoma country doctor, attended Johns Hopkins Medical School and was accepted for an internship there after he graduated in 1938. Two years later Longmire's father suffered a disabling stroke. Compelled to take over his father's practice, he gave up his coveted residency position at Hopkins. Fortunately, unable to serve in the military during World War II because of a lingering inguinal hernia, Longmire was taken back on the resident staff due to a shortage of surgical house officers. He soon fell under the creative spell of his mentor and chief, Alfred Blalock. Doctor Blalock's work with "blue babies" and innovative shunt surgery stimulated Longmire to study similar "shunt" surgery for biliary obstruction. Like many of his contemporaries, a curiosity about the biliary system spilled over to an interest in liver disease in general. His success at intrahepatic cholangiojejunostomy for recalcitrant biliary strictures prompted a certain boldness for liver surgery itself. His first hepatectomy was performed at the Johns Hopkins Hospital on October 21,

---

[9] His reputation spread far and wide. *Time* magazine would report (in a complementary tone) in 1964 that Alexander Brunschwig "has literally disemboweled hundreds of patients during the past 17 years" ("Surgery: The Most Radical Operation" *Time* July 31, 1964)

1946, for a large liver cell adenoma occupying both right and left anterior aspects of her liver. At Johns Hopkins four previous liver resections had been performed,[10] one by a youthful general surgeon named Harris Shumacker, for an hemangioma of the left lobe, and which was duly reported in 1941 [17], and three by Kenneth Pickrell and Richard Clay, after perfecting a technique for left lobectomy. In their publication 2 years after Shumacker's, the two surgeons—like others before them—acknowledged that the "cardinal objections" to resection were "severe hemorrhage" by tissue that "retains sutures so poorly" and impairment of liver function [18]. Yet, with use of full thickness mattress-type sutures, all resections had been successful.

Now 33-year-old Longmire and his 30-year-old companion Bill (H. William) Scott embarked on a rather unorthodox anterior resection utilizing the same "mattress sutures and gelatin sponges" to stave the blood loss which, with this nonanatomic resection, was in excess of 3000 mL [19]. The next eight cases he reported to the American Surgical Association in 1961 were done in Los Angeles at the new University of California Hospital at Los Angeles (now known as UCLA) [20]. His second case was a 17-year-old with a rapidly enlarging hepatocellular carcinoma originating in the right lobe but extending across the falciform ligament into the left lobe. On July 24, 1956, a rather heroic operation was attempted, resecting the entire right lobe and a portion of the left lobe. Again, with such a nonanatomic resection, blood loss was massive and incessant. Longmire reported dispassionately:

> Interlocking mattress sutures and Gelfoam were used for hemostasis but the blood loss was great; 11,000 cc. of blood were replaced … cardiac arrest occurred at the conclusion of the procedure … the patient's postoperative course was one of progressive deterioration.

The stricken patient 10 days later of liver failure, Longmire powerless to reverse the process. The small remnant liver was totally necrotic at autopsy. It was likely a devastating experience for the lanky surgeon. Longmire did not discourage, though. His interest in liver surgery endured, and he performed seven cases over the next 4 years, not more than three cases per year. Yet all survived; five resections involving only the left lobe and three of the right lobe. Still, Longmire knew the potential of these operations—of massive hemorrhage and of leaving enough liver to sustain life. His calmness during surgery no doubt belied a deep-seated anxiety about the fate of his patients. He unflappably described one close call later:

> … a rent appeared in the middle [hepatic] vein which could be controlled only by further pressure, and further dissection in this region was temporarily abandoned … due to continued blood loss it was deemed advisable … to incise the liver beyond noncrushing clamps, control the hepatic veins, and achieve hemostasis in the hepatic parenchyma …

Longmire insisted on hilar control of portal vein and hepatic artery, at times employing complete inflow occlusion for periods up to 1 h. His worry about liver damage from ischemia prompted him to even try total body hypothermia in five cases. How to divide liver tissue continued to plague him. He was not at all

---

[10] At least these were the only ones reported in the literature.

enamored with the finger-fracture method of Asian surgeons, rather preferring the mattress suture even at the expense of injuring liver tissue at the margin. "There is no doubt it is advantageous to eliminate the use of mattress sutures and their necrosing effect on the liver margin … However, we still find a place for the mattress suture in clinical practice," he would write.

Over the next decade Longmire's UCLA group would perform 26 more liver resections, averaging a mere 2–3 cases per year. In December 1973, he gave a report of his accumulated experience before the Southern Surgical Association in Hot Springs, Virginia. Twenty-one years before, almost to the day, Julian Quattlebaum had stood and delivered his "Massive Resection of the Liver" before the same group. There would be only two deaths in Longmire's series. Like his European counterparts, Longmire, the master tactician, would carefully lay out his approach and enumerate the steps in a successful hepatic resection, echoing thoughts of others: a generous incision (even into the thorax), wide mobilization of the liver, dissection and ligation of hilar vessels, division of pertinent hepatic veins, and ligation of crisscrossing biliary and vascular structures within the liver parenchyma [21].

References

1. Wangensteen OH (1951) Cancer of the esophagus and the stomach. American Cancer Society, New York, pp 92–97
2. Ariel IM (1969) George T. Pack, M.D., 1898–1969, a tribute. Am J Surg 107:443–446
3. Pack GT, Baker HW (1953) Total right hepatic lobectomy. Ann Surg 138:253–258
4. Islami AH et al (1959) Regenerative hyperplasia of the liver following major hepatectomy. Ann Surg 150:85–89
5. Pack GT et al (1962) Regeneration of human liver after major hepatectomy. Surgery 52:617–623
6. Pettinari V (1959) 41 Falle von Leberresektion. Langenbecks Arch Chir 292:540–550
7. Dagradi AB, Brearley R (1962) The surgery of hepatic tumours. Postgrad Med J 38:670–687
8. Pettinari V, Dagradi A (1963) Hepatic resection. Panminerva Med 5:123–125
9. Sarmiento JM et al (2008) Julian K. Quattlebaum, MD: American pioneer of hepatic surgery. J Am Coll Surg 207:607–611
10. Quattlebaum JK, Quattlebaum JK Jr (1959) Technique of hepatic lobectomy. Ann Surg 149:648–651
11. Hochman B, Hardy MA (2012) Richard B. Cattell: master surgeon, teacher, and innovator. J Surg Educ 69:127–131
12. Miles WE (1908) A method of performing abdomino-perineal excision for carcinoma of the rectum and of the terminal portion of the pelvic colon. Lancet 2:1812–1813
13. Cattell RB (1940) Successful removal of liver metastasis from a carcinoma of the rectum. Lahey Clin Bull 2:7–11
14. Brunschwig A (1945) Radical resections of advanced intra-abdominal cancer: summary of results of 100 patients. Ann Surg 122:923–932
15. Brunschwig A (1953) Surgery of hepatic neoplasms: with special reference to secondary malignant neoplasms. Cancer 6:725–742
16. Brunschwig A (1955) The surgery of hepatic neoplasms with special reference to right and left hepatic lobectomies. Cancer 8:1226–1233
17. Shumacker HB Jr (1942) Hemangioma of the liver. Surgery 11:209–222

18. Pickrell KL, Clay RC (1944) Lobectomy of the liver: report of three cases. Arch Surg 48:267–277
19. Longmire WP Jr, Scott HW Jr (1948) Benign adenoma of the liver: successful surgical resection of tumor involving both right and left lobes. Surgery 24:983–988
20. Longmire WP Jr, Marable SA (1961) Clinical experience with major hepatic resections. Ann Surg 154:460–473
21. Longmire WP Jr et al (1974) Elective hepatic surgery. Ann Surg 179:712–722

Chapter 9
The Anatomists

In Plato's *Dialogues*, the loquacious sage Timaeus recounts his theory of the creation of mankind thusly [1]:

> For the authors of our being, remembering the command of their father when he bade them create the human race as good as they could ... placed in the liver the seat of divination ...

And so Plato, via his mythical characters, established a vital role for the liver, presiding over all that is "happy and joyful" and "enabling it to pass the night in peace and to practice divination in sleep." There would reside the vegetative soul of man in his metaphysical world. It would be this "solid and smooth, bright and sweet" organ that would capture the imagination of anatomists for centuries to come.

Around 165 CE (Common Era) the Greek physician Galen (129–216 CE), born in the Ephesian city of Pergamon in present-day Turkey, began his greatest tome that he titled *De usu partium*, known to the world as "On the Usefulness of the Parts of the Body," an extensive description not only of anatomy but also physiology as Galen understood and interpreted his many anatomic dissections on animals, principally tailless apes, pigs, goats, and cattle. This corpus would last well over a millennium as the definitive text on anatomy and workings of the human body. In this work, Galen, in Platonian fashion, anoints the liver as one of the principal souls of man: the rational (brain), irascible (heart), and concupiscible (liver). Thus, he interpreted the liver as the seat of passion and lust, or, as Thomas Aquinas would later say, that tendency to seek the good, the tempting, the beautiful, or the desirable (For further explanation see Ref. [2]). More pertinent, perhaps, was Galen's concept of the liver as the instrument of "sanguification," the manufacturing of blood from ingested nutritive food. Chyle, he proposed, was "taken up from the stomach, altered by the flesh of the liver, and changed gradually into the nature of that flesh [blood]." It was a process akin to agitation of grapes, he postulated, the chyle "bubbling and

T. S. Helling, D. Azoulay, *Historical Foundations of Liver Surgery*,
https://doi.org/10.1007/978-3-030-47095-1_9

fermenting like new wine from the heat of the viscus and beginning to change into useful blood."[1]

In this fashion the position of the liver became critical. It seemed, at least in Galen's animal models—by extrapolation, applied to human anatomy[2]—to envelop the stomach, "clasping the liver as if by fingers"—typically five fingers (lobes)—to provide warmth for digestion of food. The liver itself, shrouded in a great tunic though it was, lay suspended from the diaphragm by "slings" to neighboring parts: the falciform ligament, the triangular ligament, and the coronary ligament. The concave surface of the liver contained the portal vein, a singular aggregation of veins from the abdominal parts that brought nutriment up to the liver. But somewhat perplexing to Galen was the distribution of the portal branches within the liver seemingly to unite again near the convex surface to form the great vena cava. His rationale: "Nature made the veins themselves in the liver the most delicate of all the veins in the whole body." Galen went on to write "[n]ature made such a great interlacement of the vessels of the liver … in order to change the nutriment completely into blood by delaying it in the viscus [liver]" [4]. It was this liver "flesh" then that conveyed its nature to the nutriments that they soon become like flesh and flow as purified blood. And from the convex surface, the large vena cava then distributed purified blood up and down to other organs of the body. As for the hepatic arteries, they bring "vital spirits" to the liver and cool its substance.

The bile, then, in Galen's physiology, was formed from residue of hepatic sanguification—basically impurities. Yellow bile flowed along the bile ducts and gallbladder into the intestine while the heavy black bile, the "thick, muddy residue" was sent to the spleen. He correctly placed the choledochus anterior to the portal vein and beside the hepatic artery and attributed the position of the gallbladder on the undersurface of the liver as pivotal in its role as excretor of impurities in the formation of blood.

Many Islamic scholars subscribed to the teachings of Galen, but were able to rescue, preserve, and disseminate Greco-Roman medical texts, particularly during the so-called Golden Islamic Age from the seventh to the fifteenth centuries. The polymath Avicenna (*Ibn-e-Sīnā*) (980–1037) wrote *Al-Qanun fii-Al-Tibb-or* (The Canon of Medicine) probably the most influential medical encyclopedia of the medieval period. In this he describes the anatomy and function of the liver, following, perhaps, teachings of Galen and, no doubt, lacking firsthand dissection of the human corpse, a practice shrouded in ambivalence for Christians and, while not explicitly forbidden by the *Qur'an* or *shari'ah* (Islamic law), likely discouraged by

---

[1] References to Galen's *De usu partium* utilized the Cornell University Press (Ithaca) two volume edition entitled *Galen: On the Usefulness of the Parts of the Body*, translated from the Greek by Margaret Tallmadge, 1968.

[2] While Galen's predecessors, Herophilus and Erasistratus of Alexandria indeed used human dissection for their anatomic portrayals in the Third Century BCE, human dissection was not permitted in the Rome of Galen's time (whether from hygienic or religious reasons is still debated). Animal models, particularly apes, in Galen's thinking, approximated human anatomy. See [3].

customary practices (*sunnah*).[3] Yet, even disregarding religious impact, few felt inclined to challenge the precepts of Galen, using his teachings as definitive dogma and seeking, through dissections (when they were done) simply to verify and not to advance anatomic knowledge. Throughout the late medieval period, the liver remained the "guardian of the breath" and seat of nutritive functions—a principal organ along with the heart, brain, and generative organs, but lacking in fibrous texture. He portrayed the liver as having a convex—abutting the diaphragm—and concave—cupping abdominal viscera—surfaces and having five lobes, a structure much more in line with carnivore models which furnished the only anatomic models available to physicians. On the undersurface hung the gallbladder connected to liver substance by a network of tributaries receiving bile from the liver and channeling it to the duodenum [6]. Of interest was Avicenna's depiction of the portal system, the *Bab*, a system that carried nutrients to the liver for formation of enriched blood. Five branches of the portal vein were represented, probably corresponding to the five-lobe Galenic lobular arrangement seen in animal genres. These all came together as minute channels to form the corresponding great vein, the vena cava that arose from the convex surface and distributed blood, via eight branches, to all the viscera [7].

The lobar structure of mammalian livers is in distinct contrast to the fused organ of humans. Henri de Mondeville (1260–1320), in the fourteenth century, ascribed to the Galenic thinking of the time and conceptualized the human liver as resembling a hand, the appendages—the term he used was "pinions"—were, as Galen had described, like the fingers of a hand, anywhere from three to five in number—perhaps referring to inferior drooping of the now recognized anterior segments (III, IV, and V). Ancient "philosophers" thought the organ resembled the liver of cattle. In de Mondeville's description—following the teachings of Galen—the human liver had a domed and a concave, furrowed surface and was closely applied to the stomach ("as if a hand held an apple," he wrote), so as to aid the stomach in its "digestive virtue." As for the complexity of veins, de Mondeville described the great "portal" vein giving forth a number of tributaries to the intestine—the mesenteric veins. The portal "capillaries" then spread throughout the substance of the liver towards the dome, in no particular fashion, to aggregate into the great vein which then emerged from the liver (inferior vena cava) which, of course, dispersed upwards and downwards. Nutritive blood was carried, in Galenic thinking, from the liver to other members of the body. Conventional wisdom considered the right ventricle of the heart the source of this elaborate venous system that ramified "as branches are borne from their trunk." As for the biliary system, the *cysta fellis*—the gallbladder—hung from the inferior surface in a membranous sac and was a reservoir of bile. Three channels emanated: one to attract bile from the liver, the second to send bile to the intestine, and a third (somewhat mysterious) channel to the stomach to strengthen digestion [8].

---

[3] A rather lengthy and comprehensive discussion of the issue of anatomic dissection in the Islamic world is found in [5].

Even the genius of Leonardo da Vinci (1452–1519) contributed. Fascinated by anatomy, da Vinci at first dissected animals to learn the intricacies of internal anatomy. Heavily influenced by Galen and Avicenna, and, no doubt, limited in his exposure to internal human anatomy, his early drawings of the liver showed five lobes, either mimicking Galen or representing nonhuman mammalian organs. In typical Galenic fashion, he wrote:

> The liver is the distributer and dispenser of nourishment vital to man. The gall bladder is the familiar servant of the liver which sweeps up and carries off all the filth and superfluities remaining after the nourishment has been distributed to all members by the liver [9].

The tributaries of the portal vein were seen by da Vinci as continuations of the hepatic vein and vena cava. Nevertheless, in 1508 da Vinci accurately drew and described the cystohepatic triangle formed by cystic artery, cystic duct and common hepatic duct, based very likely, by this time in his life, on detailed human dissection. His description predated by almost four centuries that of Jean-François Calot (1861–1944) [10].

The Flemish anatomist Andreas Vesalius (1514–1564) would revolutionize medical thinking. In *De humani corporis fabrica*, published in 1543, he correctly diagramed the liver in its familiar topographical configuration, identifying, as had his predecessors, the *cauum iecoris*—the "hollow" or concave undersurface of the organ pierced by the falciform ligament and harboring the membrane-covered gallbladder. However, he had based his anatomy on actual human dissection, a number done in Venice and Padua, at least one of which was a public demonstration in 1540 in Bologna. Here he began to depart from the traditional Galenic anatomy to which he had formerly subscribed [11]. Telling details in his *fabrica* were in stark contrast to Galen's anatomy. From posterior he drew the retrohepatic vena cava that "permeated the septum" (of the diaphragm), and traveled inferiorly, intimately associated with the liver. Further depiction of the biliary system correctly indicated that there were a system of bile channels to the right side and to the left side of the liver substance [12]. Of interest, Vesalius corrected his depiction of the liver in a previous publication of six anatomic plates, drawn by him personally and put forth as *Tabulae Anatomicae Sex* (1538). In one of these plates Vesalius directed a peculiar Galenic liver of five-lobes, seemingly radiating from a fixed central point.[4] But *De humani corporis fabrica* provided a much more faithful portrayal, even intimating an anatomic hepatic partitioning. In fact, it ranked among one of the great books of the world, so thought Sir William Osler. "It represented the full flower of the Renaissance" [13]. Yet, despite this tempting allusion to segmental liver function, Vesalius still abided by the Galenic interpretation, though, that the organ was the seat of sanguification and that veins coursing towards and away from the liver served to bring vital nutrients to liver substance and to distribute newly formed blood to other regions of the body. It would be almost a full century hence before

---

[4]These six plates were drawn by Joannes Stephanus of Calcar under the immediate direction of Vesalius and were based on his early human dissections at Padua. At the time, Vesalius was only a year out from medical school.

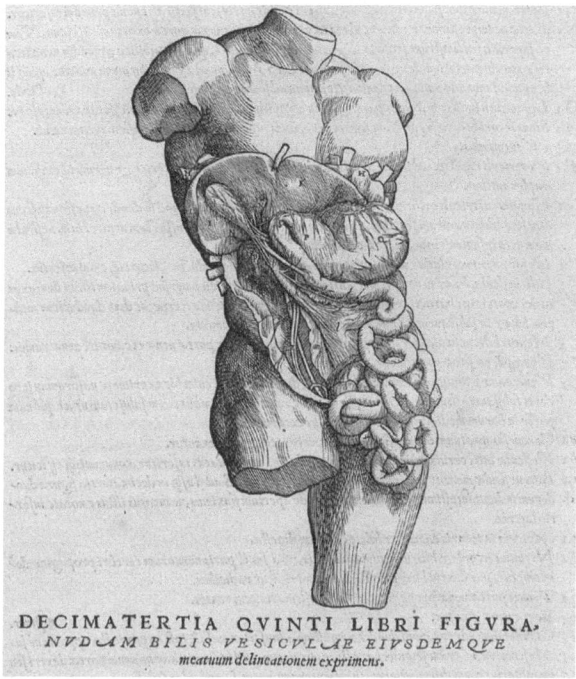

DECIMATERTIA QVINTI LIBRI FIGVRA,
*NVDAM BILIS VESICVLAE EIVSDEMQVE
meatuum delineationem exprimens.*

William Harvey detailed the arterial and venous circulations and dispelled the persistent notion that the liver was the seat of blood formation (Fig. 9.1).

The Dutch painter Gerard de Lairesse, one of the most recognized Golden Age artists after the death of Rembrandt in 1669, was commissioned by Govert Bidloo to draw life-like portraits of corpses in various stages of exposure to demonstrate, in great detail, specifics of anatomy for the text *Anatomia Humani Corporis*, eventually published in 1685. In his depiction, the painter faithfully captures detailed aspects of the topographically large right "lobe" of the liver and the accurate depiction of the undersurface, the so-called *cauum iecoris* of Vesalius. Of interest was that the faithful reproduction of Lairesse's illustrations was made possible by the use of engravings employed by Vesalius and others the century before. However, in the process of producing the copperplate Lairesse's pictures were copied in mirror image (Fig. 9.2) and published as such, creating a glaring error to educated anatomists.[5]

It feel to the Englishman Francis Glisson (1597–1677) to bring to light the inner structure of liver parenchyma and, through his detailed examinations, wonder about the segmental nature of blood flow and biliary drainage. Glisson was born in the

---

[5] Bidloo's entire work seems to have been plagiarized and published by the British anatomist William Cowper as The Anatomy of Human Bodies in 1698, but, despite protests by Bidloo, little came of it, and Cowper went on to lead a distinguished career. The entire incident is expertly chronicled by [14].

Fig. 9.2 Lairesse''s liver (left) and as it was transposed (right). In: G. Bidloo, Anatomia humani corporis (Amsterdam, 1685). BIU Santé (Paris)/ Cote ms00026

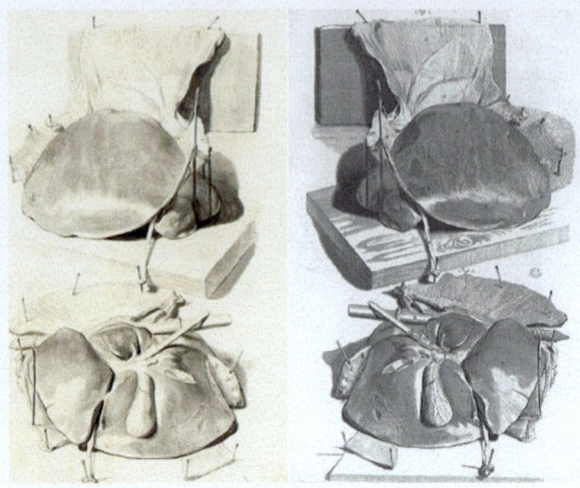

inconsequential village of Rampisham in southern England. He earned his medical degree from Cambridge in 1634, and from there "applied himself to the study of physic." His career was meteoric: member of the College of Physicians, and shortly thereafter, Regius Professor of Physic at Cambridge. Glisson became a proficient and sought-after anatomic dissector, conducting graphic demonstrations of diseased organs. In 1640, he was chosen to give the Theodore Goulston Lecture in anatomy, which he delivered in 1641. It was in preparation for this address that Glisson most likely developed the material for his opus *Anatomia Hepatis*, released in 1654 and shortly translated into Latin for wider dissemination by the scholar Sir George Ent. His preparation of the human liver for study were pioneering, "de-fleshing" the liver substance—literally cooking the liver and then teasing off parenchyma—to better elucidate internal vascular and biliary structures.[6]

In this extensive discussion, as had his predecessors, Glisson described the anatomic relationship of the liver to other abdominal viscera, detailing attachments of the liver to the diaphragm and noting the *gibbum* or "hump"—dome—of the liver. Internally, liver tissue seemed to dissolve between his fingers exposing delicate networks of veins and more substantive structures of durable connective tissue.

Glisson debated over the lobar nature of the human liver, feeling that there was a division in human liver substance, much more subtle than that seen in other animals, but not apparent on examining surface anatomy. In fact, Glisson likened the human liver, viewed from above and below, to a "hardened, cooked, egg white," more or less an oval shape as defined by its surrounding anatomy. Yet he alluded to a right and left liver "*lobos*" (lobes) defined by the falciform ligament [16]. And he acknowledged a lobe encompassing the vena cava which he termed the Spiegelian

---

[6] All further references to *Anatomia Hepatis* contained in Glisson, *Anatomia Hepatis*, (Amstelodami: Apud Joannem Janssonium a Waesberge, & Elizeum Weyerstraten, 1665). For further discussion of Glisson's tunics see [15].

lobe. The Flemish anatomist Adriaan Spiegel (1578–1625), educated in the ana-tomic mecca of Padua, had compiled a detailed anatomic text, *De humani corporis fabrica*, that, in his chapter on liver anatomy, described and termed the *duae illae eminentiae, circa venae portae egresssum locatae* (dual eminences located around the portal vein), the *lobos exiguus*, the small lobe, now, for Glisson, called Spiegel's lobe [17].

But what captured attention was Glisson's description of the internal arrange-ment of blood and biliary vessels traversing the liver bound by a common tunic that represented the enfoldings of the enveloping hepatic capsule—or, in his terms, "born of the peritoneum."

> *Ubi primum venae Portae truncum excipit, hepatis tunicae ... circumcirca continuator. Capsula enim isthaec ad cavum hepatis pertingit ... Tunica haec ramulum venae Portae comitatta ... usque pertingit, totamque illam partem ejus, quae in cavitate hepatis defoditur* (see [16], p 238).
>
> (Where first the trunk of the portal vein encounters the hepatic tunic, it is encircled and this capsule plunges into the liver ... This tunic accompanies branches of the portal vein and reaches all parts deep in the cavity of the liver)

Glisson described the portal trunk, its entry into the concave surface, and five ramifications from it through the parenchyma, not quite convinced that this repre-sented a true "lobar" arrangement, however. He also established the capillary net-work connecting fine branches of the portal system with the hepatic venous system and, ultimately, the inferior vena cava (see [16], p 224).

The Dutch physician and anatomist Isbrand van Diemerbroeck (1609–1674) gave an interesting perspective of the liver in his authoritative text *The Anatomy of Human Bodies*, written in 1672 and published in English in 1694, in which he commented

> [T]he substance of the Liver in Man consists of little Lobes, which shew forth a heap of Clusters, and are cloath'd with their own enfolding membrane ... That the whole Mass of the Liver consists of glandulous Balls and several Roots of Vessels; and hence, that they may all cooperate for the common good, there is a necessity of an intercourse between the Vessels and these Glandules [18].[7]

Van Diemerbroeck went on to describe the double venous network, the upper *Vena Cava* and lower *Vena Portae*, vessels of the liver that are "intermixed after a wonderful manner through its Substance or little Lobes" (see [18], p 81) and an interplay of branches of the portal vein which enters the liver in the hollow part (undersurface) dividing into "a thousand Branches" (see [18], p 83), all coated, of course, in Glisson's membranes. But, van Diemerbroeck admitted, how the branches of the portal vein and hepatic veins are "intermingled" was greatly disputed among anatomists of the day. He ultimately relied on the work of Glisson and the Italian microscopist Marcello Malpighi to determine that "Sanguineous humors" flowed

---

[7] Originally published in Latin as *Anatome corporis humani: plurimis novis inventis intructa* in 1672.

Fig. 9.3 Rex's drawing of
the portal venous system.
In: Rex H., Beiträge zur
Morphologie der
Säugerleber, 1888

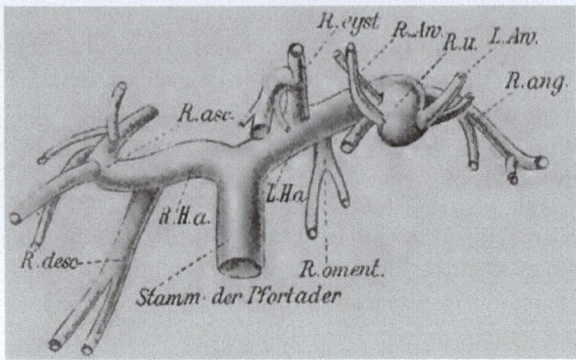

through the ends of portal vein branches into the substance of the liver and then
"sucked up through the gaping Ends of the Roots [vena cava]."[8]

So, the intertwined and complex internal arrangement of hepatic vessels and
ducts escaped attention and curiosity until the latter half of the nineteenth century
when surgeons began to challenge the intimidation of liver surgery. Hugo Rex
(1861–1936) is the informally recognized Father of Human Liver Anatomy. His
seminal work, *Beiträge zur Morphologie der Säugerleber* ("Contributions to the
Morphology of the Mammalian Liver") was published in 1888 [19]. While focusing
on other mammals, he made some startling conclusions about human anatomy.
Using corrosive casts, Rex demonstrated the primary and secondary divisions of the
portal vein in man and the regional network of vessels, not according to topographical anatomy, but distributed to right and left sides by a plane passing through the
gallbladder fossa, not falciform ligament. The distribution of secondary portal
branches on the right side further subdivided the "right liver" into a posterior (supplied by the *rechtes arcuatus et descendens* vessels) and anterior (supplied by the
rechtes ascendens vessels). The left portal vein, he noted, contained *rechtes astwerk*
(right branches) and *linkes astwerk* (left branches) to medial and lateral regions on
either side of the falciform ligament and umbilical sulcus, establishing in his mind,
the true nature of human hepatic segmentation. In fact, he described the course of
the left portal vein paralleling the umbilical sulcus giving off branches medially and
laterally. This was a radical departure from conventional thinking and placed the
essence of lobar distribution not on the liver's surface but deep within, the only
topographical landmark being the gallbladder and an imaginary plane each surgeon
must visualize. It would certainly not be an easy sell. But only as later work verified
his observations was he afforded the central place in liver anatomy that he holds
today (Fig. 9.3).

---

[8] Van Diemerbroeck, *The Anatomy of Human Bodies*, 83; Marcello Malpighi meticulously
described the microscopic anatomy of the liver in man, defining the hexagonal glandular nature
organized as "acini", involved in manufacturing bile, but could not identify direct connections of
the portal and vena cava circulation (*Marcello Malphighi e L'opera Sua*, [Milan: Francesco
Vallardi, Ed, 1897], 118–119).

It is sometimes providence that advances the fortunes of man. So it may have been with Sir James Cantlie (1851–1926). He was of Scottish origin, born in Dufftown, Banffshire in 1851. Mitchell Bruce, a lifelong friend, described him as a lad with a "confident countenance, and hearty, kindly, straightforward manner."[9] He received his degree in arts and medicine from the University of Aberdeen. He then left for London where he completed his medical studies at Charing Cross Hospital. It was here that he developed an interest in anatomy and, in fact, was appointed a demonstrator of anatomy in the school. In 1877, Cantlie became the assistant surgeon to the hospital and was admitted to the Royal College of Surgeons. But the young surgeon-anatomist had a *wanderlust* not satiated by local travel. Perhaps it was fueled by a trip to Egypt in 1883 to help with an outbreak of cholera—a developing fascination with the East. Ten years later he was off to the *Far* East—China—relinquishing his post as house surgeon, perhaps encouraged by the harsh criticism he received after delivering a scathing diatribe on London life entitled "*Degeneration Amongst Londoners*" in 1885.[10]

His visit to Hong Kong was at the invitation of another Aberdeen graduate, Sir Patrick Manson, the first Dean of the Hong Kong College of Medicine. It was in Hong Kong that Cantlie came across that Chinese prisoner who had hanged himself in jail. His postmortem provided an impetus for Cantlie to rethink conventional concepts of liver anatomy. The right side of this man's liver (not "lobe" as Cantlie pointed out) was a mass of fibrous tissue from a liver abscess, the right portal vein, artery, and duct all obliterated. Hypertrophy of the left side was the consequence. But what drew Cantlie's attention was that the hypertrophy involved Spiegel's lobe—"*lobules spigelii*"—(the left part of the caudate lobe) and the quadrate lobe (essentially the left medial section), two areas of the liver normally attributed to the right lobe. He then performed his experiments. Dividing the liver through the plane of the gallbladder fossa towards the inferior vena cava gave portions that were almost identical in weight—"within a few ounces, sometimes a drachm or two." The primary branches of the portal vein, hepatic artery, and bile ducts are "practically of the same size." Injecting the right and left divisions of the portal vein with different colored agents demonstrated a separation plane through the gallbladder fossa to the inferior vena cava, the same plane he used to cleave the liver. The injections produced little if any crossover. Clinically speaking, he noted that the liver, when traumatized "as between the buffers of railway-carriages, splits along the mid-line of the liver [the same gallbladder plane] in preference to any other." In his thinking, this lent symmetry to the human liver and afforded surgeons the opportunity to work in a relatively bloodless plane. Cantlie was convinced that if surgeons were to follow his recommendations "the surgery of the liver will be advanced a step." It only awaited clinical confirmation:

---

[9] From an obituary published in the *British Medical Journal* for June 5, 1926 (no author), 971–972.

[10] This was a lecture delivered at the Parkes Museum of Hygiene on January 27, 1885 in which he attacked the urban environment of London as distinctly unhealthy from the lack of fresh air to the absence of sunshine to the inability to exercise [20].

The practical bearing of this [the plane through the gallbladder fossa—"Cantlies's line"] has yet to be proved surgically; but there can be no doubt that any surgical interference with the liver will be much more readily tolerated as it approaches that line, which I have termed the mid-line of the liver, and that the haemorrhage has less to be dreaded as the liver is incised or torn in the neighbourhood of that line (Quotes from [21]).

But surgery of the liver was not James Cantlie's passion. Instead, he devoted much of his career to the study of tropical diseases, a constant concern in the far-flung British Empire. He was soon appointed Dean of the Hong Kong College of Medicine, replacing Sir Patrick Manson. He returned to London in 1897 and founded what eventually became the London School of Tropical Medicine. But his major accomplishment was work he did during the First World War in educating British troops on the new concept of "first aid," becoming an Honorary Colonel in the Royal Army Medical Corps Training. His advice on initial care of the wounded was a novel concept that may have saved life and limb of countless men in the trenches "far from surgical help." Never again, though, did he write about the liver or, for any intents and purposes, operate on this fascinating organ. He died in his 75th year after a long illness, apparently never the light-hearted man after the untimely death of his beloved wife, Lady Mabel Cantlie. And never in his lifetime would he be acknowledged for his pivotal, if obscure, contribution to liver surgery (Fig. 9.4).

It was not until the 1920s, a generation later, that Cantlie's work was brought to light through the efforts of two Mayo Clinic physicians, Archibald McIndoe (1900–1960) and Virgil Counseller (1892–1977). McIndoe was a native of New Zealand, born in Dunedin on the South Island in 1900. He completed his medical training at the University of Otago and became a house surgeon at Waikato Hospital in Hamilton on the North Island. His break came with a visit by Will Mayo, who, during a tour of the University of Otago, offered a fellowship to a graduate of the school. McIndoe was the lucky recipient. He was off to Rochester, Minnesota. As First Assistant in Pathological Anatomy, he teamed up with a young Mayo surgeon, Virgil Counseller from Illinois, in studies on the liver. There had been a flurry of reports, mostly French, alluding to the separate circulation of the two halves of the

Fig. 9.4 Cantlie's line demarcating right and left livers. Cantlie J., Proc Anat Soc Great Britain, 1897

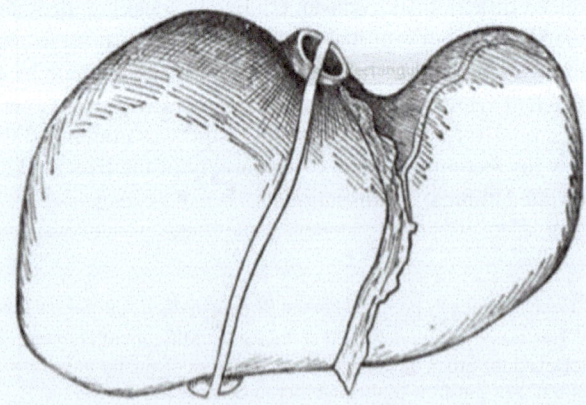

liver, and, more or less, supporting Cantlie's observations. The liver of man was held to be a fused organ. Yet, where was the line of demarcation? McIndoe and Counseller injected a series of human livers with different color celloidins and found a "striking and constant result." Left and right branches of the portal vein, hepatic artery, and bile duct demonstrated a line of division extending through the gallbladder fossa obliquely towards the entrance of the hepatic veins into the inferior vena cava and splitting the caudate lobe cleanly in half. Their anatomic findings confirmed the rather informal experiments of Cantlie—that the liver is divided into two equal parts not by the falciform ligament but by the gallbladder—Cantlie's line [22]. In fact, the two scientists illustrated Rex's arborialization of the portal system with its secondary ramifications. Despite further work describing surgery for hepatocellular carcinoma (and a rather notable—and successful—operation on gangster Al Capone's younger brother), McIndoe left the Mayo Clinic after 5 years for England, developing a surgical practice there and becoming deeply involved in burn care for wounded pilots of the Royal Air Force in World War II. His contributions to plastic surgery earning him knighthood in 1947 would far outweigh, in notoriety, his discoveries in liver anatomy.

But then, one must not forget the contributions of that obscure Vietnamese physician by the name of Tôn Thất Tùng, who, with unbridled energy and enthusiasm, dissected hundreds of livers in the exotic Indochinese city of Hà Nội to find an answer to that ubiquitous Vietnamese problem of ascariasis. In the process Tùng, without any prior knowledge of the works of Rex or Cantlie, unraveled the deep mysteries of liver anatomy. By using delicate injection methods, Tùng delineated portal and venous networks of veins, two distinct venous systems, regional in their distribution. These studies he used as the basis for his doctoral thesis *La Vascularisation Veineuse du Foie et ses Applications aux Résections et Lobectomies Hépatiques* ("The Venous Vascularization of the Liver and its Application for Hepatic Resections and Lobectomies") published in 1935 in the first volume of proceedings of the Anatomic Institute of the Indochinese Medical School in Hanoi (*Institut Anatomique de l'École Supérieure de Médecine de l'Indochine*) and later, in 1939, as his completed thesis and first book-length publication. However, his discoveries would not be recognized globally until long after the publications of western anatomists.[11]

Carl-Herman Hjortsjö (1914–1978) was born in Malmo, Sweden. He was the son of a physician, Herold Hirschlaff. Like his father, young Carl decided on a similar path, but his career would be one of the anatomic sciences. He graduated from the University of Lund, focusing on anatomy. His graduate thesis was on the early morphogenesis of epithelial pulmonary primordium in the cat. However, his interests broadened to include anthropology and paleopathology, participating in a number of international archeological expeditions. Together with the zoologist Nils-Gustaf Gejvall, he established the Swedish Expedition for Archaeological Anthropology in

---

[11] For reference see Refs. [23] and [24]. See also a more detailed review of Tùng's anatomic work in Ref. [25].

1951. He made significant contributions to historical research from his anthropo-
logical studies of the remains of historical figures, including the Swedish Saint
Birgitta of Vadstena, one of the six patron saints of Europe. It was the study of her
skeletal remains that prompted Hjortsjö to speculate whether she suffered from epi-
lepsy rather than the spiritual ecstasies that she claimed to endure. He went on to
head the Institute of Anatomy in Lund.

In 1947, Hjortsjö began studying intrahepatic anatomy, focusing on the biliary
system. He made a series of corrosion specimens of the portal veins and used a lead-
based dye, injecting the bile ducts and hepatic arteries so that radiographs could be
obtained with the liver in situ. The results were startling. The corrosion specimens
showed a clear division by a "main boundary fissure" into right and left "halves."
The avascular fissure did not correspond to the falciform ligament or umbilical fissure. It cut obliquely through the liver in the fashion described by Cantlie and con-
formed precisely to his "plane." Moreover, on the right side fissures also subdivided
the region into three parts, which Hjortsjö termed dorso-caudal, intermediate, and
ventro-cranial segments. The left region seemed subdivided into medial and lateral
portions. His stereoscopic radiographs of the biliary system were remarkable in
their clarity. However, his main boundary fissure was not as apparent, the right and
left ducts projecting on each other, due largely to the slanted course of the fissure
and the angle of the X-ray beam. Correlating corrosion specimens and cholangio-
grams, Hjortsjö was able to conclude that portal vein and duct accompanied one
another in pedicle fashion. His studies were finally published in 1951 [26]. Once
again, in conclusive fashion, the segmental nature of blood flow and bile drainage of
the human liver was demonstrated, even down to sectional territories. Yet another
patch in the mosaic of hepatic anatomy was stitched into place.

Enter Claude Couinaud (1922–2008). Former President of the Americas Hepato-
Pancreato-Biliary Association, Jean-Nicholas Vauthey, puts him at the crossroads of
development of hepatic surgery, a key figure in launching liver surgery into a new
dimension [27]. Couinaud was born in the Norman town of Argentan, near the Orne
River. It was a community known for metal and food industries, growing to a population over 7000 by the eve of World War II. But the war would sweep over it. Like
so many Normandy villages, Argentan was engulfed and destroyed in the Allied
invasion of 1944. By then the young Couinaud had already left, beginning his medical studies in Paris in 1940. Upon graduation in 1946 he started his surgical training,
completing it in 1951. He then studied for 3 months with the brilliant thoracic surgeon, Professor Phillip Allison in Leeds, England. It was here that he was introduced to the field of anatomy and its application to surgery, delving into the
segmental distribution of intrapulmonary vasculature. Upon return to France, at the
age of 30 he was awarded a *Professeur Agrégé* to study with the renowned anatomist
André Delmas at the University of Paris.[12] Professor Delmas encouraged his young

---

[12]André Delmas (1910–1999) had become *Chef des Travaux Anatomiques* of the Faculty of
Medicine of Paris in 1947 (the last professor to hold that title). He stressed the importance of
detailed dissection, integrating topographical anatomy with internal pathways and function (he
himself concentrated on cranial anatomy). For further information see Ref. [28].

pupil to focus on liver anatomy. Couinaud, at the suggestion of Delmas, employed a technique that he developed to "cast" the intrahepatic vasculature and biliary system using hardened polyvinyl acetate. The liver parenchyma was then dissolved around the cast, giving a detailed representation of the distribution of vessels and bile ducts. By 1952, he began to recognize a territorial arrangement of liver blood flow and biliary drainage, much as suggested by Rex and Cantlie a half century before (he did not mention the far away Annamite surgeon/anatomist Tung, who stumbled onto similar conclusions in the 1930s). At this point he returned to clinical surgery as *Chef de Clinique* for the celebrated *Professeur* Henri Mondor.[13]

Yet Couinaud's anatomic work did not cease—clinical duties in the mornings and casting, examining, recording in the afternoons [30]. He would eventually accumulate well over 100 liver casts for determining the course of intraparenchymal structures. In 1952, he published the first description of his interpretation of hepatic anatomy focusing on the *parenchyme à gauche* and its segmental blood supply. By this time he had already suggested nomenclature for his system of veins and arteries, defining the left liver by segments II, III, and IV. In doing so, he distinguished the "classic" left lobectomy (segments II and III) from a true, or total, left hepatectomy incorporating segment IV as well, and centering on a hilar approach for definition of right and left "lobes" [31]. In this description he incorporated the "Glissonean" capsule in encircling and controlling hepatic inflow. At the time of his publication he was but 30 years old, just embarking on his surgical career, but with a clearer understanding of liver anatomy than most of his contemporaries or, for that matter, his masters. In 1954, he formalized his interpretation of intrahepatic anatomy in an article published in *Presse Medicale* entitled *Lobes et Segments Hepatiques* [32]. By that time his report was based on 120 liver casts and 50 dissections of fresh organs. Referring to the work of Hugo Rex decades past, he correlated his findings with those of the German anatomist, proposing four regions of the liver—he termed these *territoires*—two comprising the right liver and two the left. These regions received a Glissonean pedicle and were separated by one of the three hepatic veins. He named them *territoires medial* and *lateral* (*partie gauche*) and *territoires lateroinférieur* and *centro-supérieur* comprising *partie droite*.[14] And he went on to suggest "*Ces quatre territoires hépatiques peuvent être scindés en un certain nombre de segments*" (these four liver territories can be divided into some number of segments), the basis for his segmental anatomy. How did Couinaud come up with his segment numbering system? "It all came from Rex," he told his interviewers Jean Vauthey and Eddie Abdalla in 2000. To him Rex played the pivotal role in defining liver anatomy[15] (Fig. 9.5).

---

[13] Henri Mondor (1885–1962) was an icon of French surgery. Eclectic in his pursuits, Mondor developed expertise in rectal cancer, gynecologic surgery, emergency surgery, not to mention his passion for literature, art, and history. See the article by Ober [29].

[14] The right hepatic vein separated the *centro-superieur* territory (segments V and VIII) from the *latero-inferieur* territory (segments VI and VII); the middle hepatic vein separated the *partie droite* from *partie gauche*; and the left hepatic vein separated *territoires medial and lateral*.

[15] Vauthey, et al. "From Couinaud to Molecular Biology".

Fig. 9.5 Schematic of
Couinaud's liver segments.
From Couinaud C., La
Presse Medicale, 1954

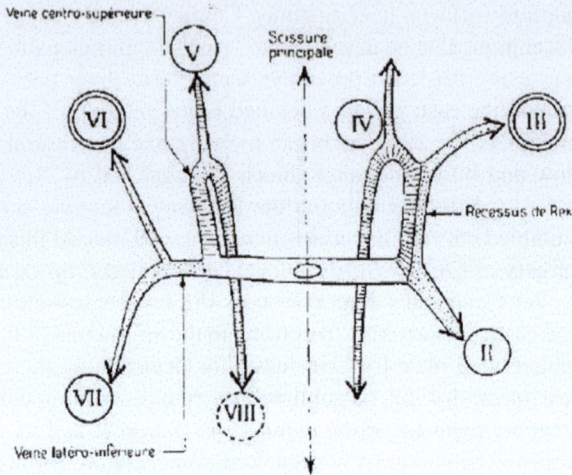

In fact, calling upon the work of McIndoe and Counseller who had proposed two distinct halves to the liver, one almost mirroring the other, Couinaud followed the lead of Laux and Rapp and their theory of symmetry presented at the *Société Anatomique* in July 1953. These anatomists diagramed halves of the liver containing identical superior and posterior sectional branches of the portal vein [33]. Couinaud went further, identifying two segments supplied by each portal branch (the superior branch on the left supplying anterior and posterior parts of segment IV). This represented a true symmetry to the liver, his "*symetrie du foie*": the superior section (segments V and VIII) and inferior section (segments VI and VII) on the right that mirrored the superior (segment IV) and inferior (segments II and III) sections on the left. His conclusion was that "*il existe une symétrie particulièrement frappante entre les deux foies dans la disposition segmentaire et dans la distribution des pédiculés portes*" ("there is a particularly striking symmetry between the two livers in segmental disposition and distribution of portal pedicles"). Yet he acknowledged that there was great variability in human livers, the right usually, but not always, predominating. Even still, the umbilical scissura and falciform ligament would continue to stymie anatomic purists. Symmetry was better visualized on paper rather than in vivo, running directly underneath giving branches to the three segments in a fashion not nearly as clean as the right liver.

Ken Takasaki, surgeon at the Tokyo Women's Medical University, revolutionized the thinking about liver segmentation by introducing, in 1986, the concept of three secondary portal pedicle branchings, each supplying, in his estimation, about 30 percent of the liver substance (the smaller caudate branchings account for the remaining 10%). These he termed the right sector (Couinaud's segments VI and VII), the middle sector (Couinaud's segments V and VIII), and the left sector (Couinaud's segments II, III, and IV). Takasaki's anatomy takes into account the early (or completely nonexistent) branching of the "right" portal pedicle so that two of his three pedicles supply the "right" liver (anterior and posterior sectors) and the third, the "left" liver. So, in a sense, Takasaki was describing a trilobed liver. Ramifications of his Glissonean pedicles are located just outside the portal surface of the liver. Control of these pedicles, encompassing the entire Glissonean structures (he has shown they are the same extrahepatic and intrahepatic) extrahepatically, is thus possible for selective hepatic resections that he termed *systematized hepatectomy*.[16] Takasaki used this method to resect hepatocellular carcinoma with preservation of the maximum amount of liver tissue yet incorporating all branches of the portal system supplying the tumor, and, in fact, has been embraced by Vietnamese surgeons in Hà Nội [35].[17] Is this in conflict with Couinaud's "holy grail" of segmental liver anatomy? Professor Henri Bismuth, who wrote the Foreword for Takasaki's textbook, felt not:

> We can say that portal blood is distributed to three portions of the liver: the right segment, the middle segment, and the left segment for Takasaki, and the right posterior sector, the right anterior sector, and the left liver for Couinaud. Thus the liver is divided into three in both classifications [36].[18]

In other words, Takasaki and Couinaud were in agreement. The segmental and sectoral nature of liver anatomy would stand as a guide to territorial approaches to liver surgery. It was through the genius of these two anatomists, perched on the works of others before them, that a rational interpretation of the inner domains of such a mysterious organ had finally been brought to light.

References

1. Plato (1892) The dialogues of Plato: republic, Timaeus, Critias, translated by B. Jowett. Macmillan, London
2. Miner R (2009) Thomas Aquinas on the passions: a study of summa Theologiae. Cambridge University Press, Cambridge, pp 56–58
3. Conner A (2017) Galen's analogy: animal experimentation and anatomy in the second century C.E. Anthós 8:118–145
4. Tallmadge M (1968) Galen: on the usefulness of the parts of the body. Cornell University Press, Ithaca
5. Savage-Smith E (1995) Attitudes toward dissection in medieval Islam. J Hist Med Allied Sci 50:67–110

---

[16] Bernard Launois from the University of Rennes had described a similar Glissonean approach to resection in 1992 but it must be remembered that Takasaki described it first some 6 years before [34].

[17] The author (TSH) has personally observed a rather systematized approach to segmental liver resection using Takasaki's approach by surgeons at the Viet Duc University Hospital in Hanoi.

[18] Ken Takasaki was much admired in his homeland of Japan. In the Forward for his text, Masatoshi Makuuchi wrote of him "I am devoted to Professor Takasaki because he is a true liver surgeon, a man of few words, with a sharp mind and excellent hands" (Takasaki, *Glissonean Pedicle Transection*, viii). Takasaki was a prolific surgeon, performing almost 4000 liver resections in his career.

6. Mazengenya P, Bhikha R (2018) Revisiting Avicenna's (980-1037 AD) anatomy of the abdominal viscera from the canon of medicine. Morphologie 102:225–230
7. Heydari MD et al (2018) The concept of portal system obstruction in Avicenna's canon of medicine. Acta Med Hist Adriat 16:115–126
8. Nicaise E (1893) Chirurgie de Maitre Henri de Mondeville. Felix Alcan, Paris, pp 71–72
9. O'Malley CD (1952) Leonardo da Vinci on the human body. Henry Schuman, New York, p 414
10. Calot F (1891) De la Cholecystectomie (Ablation de la Vesicule Biliaire). G. Steinheil, Paris, p 41, [doctoral thesis]
11. Lanska D (2015) The evolution of Vesalius' perspective on Galen's anatomy. Istoriya Meditsiny 2:13–26
12. Vesalius A (1555) De Humani Corporis Fabrica. Joannes Oporinus, Brussels, pp 618–622
13. Osler SW (1921) The evolution of modern medicine. Yale University Press, New Haven, p 154
14. Guest, Margocsy, Wigmore (2014) The art of medicine: Govert Bidloo's liver: human symmetry reflected. Lancet 383:688–689
15. Helling TS, McCleary SP (2016) The tunics of Glisson. Surgery 160:94–99
16. Glisson F (1665) Anatomia hepatis. Joanne Jansson, Amsterdam, p 101
17. van den Spiegel A (1632) De Humani Corporis Fabrica Libri Decem, Venice. Self-published, p 302
18. Van Diemerbroeck I (1694) The anatomy of human bodies, comprehending the most modern discoveries and curiosities. W. Whitwood, London, p 79
19. Rex H (1888) Beitrage zur Morphologie der Saugerleber. Wilhelm Engelmann, Leipzig
20. Cantlie J (1885) Degeneration amongst Londoners. Field & Tuer, London, pp 7–61
21. Cantlie J (1897) On a new arrangement of the right and left lobes of the liver. Proc Anat Soc Great Britain:iv–ix
22. McIndoe AH, Counseller VS (1927) The bilaterality of the liver. Arch Surg 1:971–972
23. Huard P et al (1937) Anatomie Chirurgicale du Foie. Travaux de l'Institut Anatomique de l'Ecole Superieure de Medecine de l'Indochine. Tome 1, Hanoi
24. Tùng TT (1939) La Vascularisation Veineuse du Foie et ses Applications aux Resections et Lobectomies Hepatique. G. Taupin & Cie, Hanoi
25. Helling TS, Azoulay D (2014) Ton that Tung's livers. Ann Surg 259:1245–1252
26. Hjortsjo C (1951) The topography of the intrahepatic duct systems. Acta Anat (Basel) 11:599–615
27. Vauthey J-N et al (2012) From Couinaud to molecular biology: the seven virtues of hepato-pancreato-biliary surgery. HPB 14:493–499
28. Saban R (2000) André Delmas (1910-1999). Hist Sci Med 34:187–188
29. Ober WB (1972) Henri Mondor [1885-1962]. NY State J Med 72:2222–2227
30. Sutherland FH et al (2002) Claude Couinaud: a passion for the liver. Arch Surg 137:1305–1310
31. Couinaud C (1952) Hepatectomies Gauches Lobaires et Segmentaires. J Chir 68:697–715
32. Couinaud C (1954) Lobes et Segments Hepatique: Notes sur l'Architecture Anatomique et Chirurgicale du Foie. Presse Med 62:709–712
33. Laux G, Rapp PE (1953) Le Dispositif Veineux du Lobe de Spiegel. CR Assoc Anat 78:264–272
34. Launois BJ (1992) The importance of Glisson's capsule and its sheaths in the intrahepatic approach to resection of the liver. Surg Gynecol Obstet 174:7–10
35. Takasaki KK et al (1986) Highly selected hepatic resection by Glisson sheath-binding method. Dig Surg 3:121
36. Takasaki K (2007) Glissonean pedicle transection method for hepatic resection. Springer, Tokyo

Chapter 10
The French School

French surgeons would have a major impact on liver and biliary tract surgery, not only in anatomic clarification but also in clinical practice. The French School,[1] or, more specifically, Paris medicine, arose from the ashes of the *ancien régime* and on the heels of the French Revolution at the turn of the nineteenth century. Departing from eighteenth century theories and systems, French physicians, with a sudden wealth of clinical material brought about by a new and entitled public hospital system, focused on clinical observation, vivisection, and intense scrutiny of abundant autopsy cases. According to Ann La Berge and Caroline Hannaway the medical practices of Paris were characterized by a correlation of clinical observations with pathological anatomy, a vast supply of patients, and concentration not just on patient history but also physical examination brought about by new and exciting diagnostic methods. The hospital now became the center of clinical activity and research. And, importantly, surgery and medicine were unified, surgeons attaining the same rank and prestige, finally, as their medical colleagues and counterparts[2]. The medical community, in the words of George Weisz, was "a huge, interlinked, and prestigious network" of municipal hospitals and several hundred physicians and surgeons [1]. Renowned researchers and experimentalists such as Francois Magendie and Claude Bernard advanced French pathology and physiology to the forefront of European

---

[1] The "French School" here pertains to the aggregate effort of (mostly) Parisian academic surgeons to detail and report their clinical experiences through professional organizations such as the highly respected *Académie de chirurgie*, a forum for *professeurs* of the Paris School of Medicine to present and discuss clinical topics.

[2] See an in-depth discussion of changes brought about by the French Revolution in Matthew Ramsey "From Expert to Spécialiste: The Conception of Specialization in Eighteenth- and Nineteenth-Century French Surgery" in *History of Ideas in Surgery: Proceedings of the 17th International Symposium for the Comparative History of Medicine* [Yosio Kawakita, ed], (Shizuoka: Ishiyaku EuroAmerica, 1992), 69–117.

T. S. Helling, D. Azoulay, *Historical Foundations of Liver Surgery*, https://doi.org/10.1007/978-3-030-47095-1_10

medical science, an *élan scientifique* in the words of Jules Rochard in his treatise *Histoire de la chirurgie français au XIXe siècles* written in 1875[3] .

By the 1830s surgical specialization was well entrenched in Paris, according to medical historian Georg Weisz, a coming together of three important requisites: (1) the unification of medicine and surgery; (2) the rapid expansion of knowledge, particularly in anatomy, pathology, and, soon, physiology; and (3) institutional changes that allowed for the focused practice of surgery on similar types of patients [2]. By 1862 42% of all practitioners in Paris were labeled as "surgeons" [3]. It was on sound anatomic foundations that surgery flourished in late-nineteenth-century Paris. One individual who revolutionized anatomical instruction was Louis Hubert Farabeuf (1841–1910). Admitted to the Faculty of Medicine of Paris in 1876, he had been trained as surgeon and anatomist. Under his direction the teaching of anatomy was radically redesigned. The classrooms were organized from beginner level to advanced study, spacious and well ventilated; the use of cadavers was expanded with injection of preserving agents to lessen the odor; and instructors and prosectors were carefully chosen and personally supervised. Farabeuf himself would often attend the dissections, relentlessly quizzing the students and pointing out subtle aspects of anatomy. His publications of operative surgery, his *Précis de Manuel Opératoire* written in three volumes became very popular, of pocket-size so as to be widely used, including by doctors at the front during World War I.[4] Even in 1955 René Leriche was said to have declared that Farabeuf had a decisive influence on French surgery [4].

Farabeuf's influence was far-reaching. It was through his tutelage that a young Uruguayan named Lorenzo Merola (1880–1935) traveled to Paris and studied abdominal anatomy, particularly that of the liver. He then returned to his native Montevideo at the Pasteur Hospital and in 1919 published a description of the peritoneal attachments of the right lobe of the liver and techniques necessary for mobilization of the right lobe by dividing these attachments [5]. Subsequently he perfected an operative approach to the dome of the liver via a thoraco-abdominal incision, through the tenth intercostal space and across the costal cartilage exposing both the pleural and peritoneal cavities [6]. In a later article Merola described the suspensory peritoneal attachments anchoring the liver in the right upper abdomen.

It was Merola's intense interest in the liver that fueled one of his bright pupils, Gerardo Caprio (1902–1977) to focus on liver surgery at the Pasteur Hospital. By virtue of the anatomic teachings of his master Caprio performed the first (topographic) left hepatic lobectomy in 1929 for a metastatic deposit of melanoma and reported his feat to the Surgery Society of Uruguay in 1931. In his presentation Caprio freely mentioned that undertaking such a momentous operation was only made possible by the lessons learned from Merola. Mimicking the great anatomist, Caprio detailed his operative approach to the audience describing his mobilization

---

[3] Taken largely from *Constructing Paris Medicine* edited by Caroline Hannaway and Ann La Berge, Editions Rodopi B.V., Amsterdam, 1998, pp. 1–71.

[4] The *Précis* did not address visceral surgery as the entire specialty was in its infancy and poorly codified during the final decades of the Nineteenth Century.

of the left lobe by dividing the left triangular ligament, and then splitting paren-chyma about 1 cm from the suspensory ligament using only three catgut sutures, one each for what we now call the Glissonean pedicles to segments II and III and then the left hepatic vein. In all this, little blood was spilt, he touted. Caprio then informed his listeners that regeneration would restore liver mass, the whole process completed within 3 or 4 weeks [7]. There was mixed reaction to his achievement. Some older surgeons felt he was promoting "surgical acrobatics" and that liver resection had no future [8].

And then Paris medicine received another boost. *Ordonnance* 50.1373 issued on December 30, 1958, created university and hospital collaboration that allowed the integration of basic and clinical science and interaction of research, teaching, and patient care—basically anointing a full-time Faculty of Medicine. The formal cre-ation of the *Assistance publique-Hôpitaux de Paris* (AP-HP) cemented the mission of providing care for the poor, the elderly, and the incurable. In part this may have been due to the reorganization of the public hospital system in France. Prior to 1958 medical education and medical care were distinctly separate. No formal links existed. The *assistance publique* established as far back as King Francois I in 1544 and consolidated under Napoleon III in 1849 placed governance of hospitals in the hands of the central government rather than municipalities.[5] By mid-nineteenth cen-tury the system was enormous encompassing 26 hospitals and in excess of 22,000 beds (although many wretchedly ventilated). Twenty-six professors, composing the *Faculté de Médecine* exerted absolute power, answering to no one but the govern-ment. Under them were 24 *agrégés*, or who would be called associate or vice-professors awaiting vacancies at the top to ascend in their academic and clinical careers [9]. It was generally considered among Americans anyway, that in medicine and surgery "France stands *first*" with a better regulated hospital system and system for medical education (quotes from [9]). However, by the twentieth century the system was in serious need of reform. There was a chronic shortage of beds, failing to keep up with urban demographics, particularly in Paris, bordering on scandalous reports.

With such a vast and academically minded initiative, the bringing together of basic scientists and clinicians enhanced and accelerated work in anatomy, physiol-ogy, and technology. But it was this reform in 1958 that brought university and hospital together as a single entity:

> The hospital presents as a center of innovation in which advanced medicine is practiced, and it is this aspect that attracts the sick of the upper classes … especially at the level of the University Hospital Centers [10].

---

[5] Practically speaking the *assistance publique* had its true beginnings with the French Revolution. At that juncture, health delivery throughout Paris radically changed and was placed in secular hands and out of control of the monarchy and Catholic Church. Beginning with the nineteenth century, a spirit of inquisitiveness and experimentalism swept the medical community, encouraged by sweeping changes in governance of public health following the French Revolution.

They were enormous facilities, dwarfing anything to date in the United States. By the 1850s *Hôpital Saint-Louis*, built at the beginning of the seventeenth century, hosted 853 beds, *La Charité* 494 beds, the ancient *Hôtel Dieu* 810 beds, and the former gunpowder factory, *Hôpital Pitié-Salpêtrière*, 624 beds. They were devoted to teaching as well, each hospital containing an amphitheater for didactic and patient-oriented teaching (figures from [9]). Some had even specialized, focusing on such areas as dermatology and gynecology.

Considering the scope of public service, it was the French who would propel liver surgery to the forefront. The crux was an understanding of liver anatomy, at least a working knowledge of anatomy that would lend itself to surgical approaches. The great French liver surgeons of the 1960s and 1970s were the products of a wealth of French surgical talent that developed in the post-war years and a lineage of facile and flamboyant gastrointestinal surgeons. Lortat-Jacob, the famous pioneer of hepatic resection, was, himself, a "visceral" surgeon, more interested, actually, in surgery of the esophagus and stomach.

Two key surgeons led the way in digestive surgery. Antonin Gosset (1872–1944), chief surgeon at the venerable *Hôpital Pitié-Salpêtrière*, focused on digestive diseases, not just liver or biliary tract. Gosset himself was the son of a physician entering the University of Paris and its School of Medicine in 1889 at the age of 17 under the tutelage of Theodore Tuffier (1857–1929), the preeminent French surgeon of his time, and becoming *chef de service* in 1912. The distinguished Gosset had written extensively about war wounds of the abdomen and head from his experiences in World War I, but his principle contributions were on surgery for cancer and surgery of the biliary tract. During his illustrious career Professor Gosset would train 100 "assistants" who would populate the hospitals of Paris and write with their mentor the seminal text of the day "*Techniques Chirurgicales*" based on experiences at the *Salpêtrière*. André Bergeret (1884–1969), a true task-master and demanding technician, presided over a stable of skilled gastrointestinal surgeons in training distributed across Paris but most notably at the *Hôpital Saint-Antoine*. Bergeret, himself a student of the flamboyant and brusque Henri Hartmann (1860–1952), had developed a vast surgical practice, spanning clinics and hospitals throughout Paris. Some of his pupils, because of his inspiration, dove into the mysteries of liver and bile ducts. Bergeret's style was a matter of master and apprentice, eager young surgeons vying for a place at the table of their teacher, year after year, until they, too, when opportunity presented, were anointed *chef de clinique* or *chirurgien des hôpitaux*. Little inclined to conversation during his cases, Bergeret expected undivided attention, demanding that his acolytes watch each move done again and again until the student, by sheer repetition, mastered the procedure. Bergeret would maintain an impeccable reputation throughout his career and publish widely, his works consistently concise without the boring, self-aggrandizing rhetoric found in so many papers of the times.[6]

---

[6] For an interesting summation of Bergeret's life and career see [11].

Fig. 10.1 Jacques Hepp.
BIU Santé (Paris)/Cote
CIPB1914

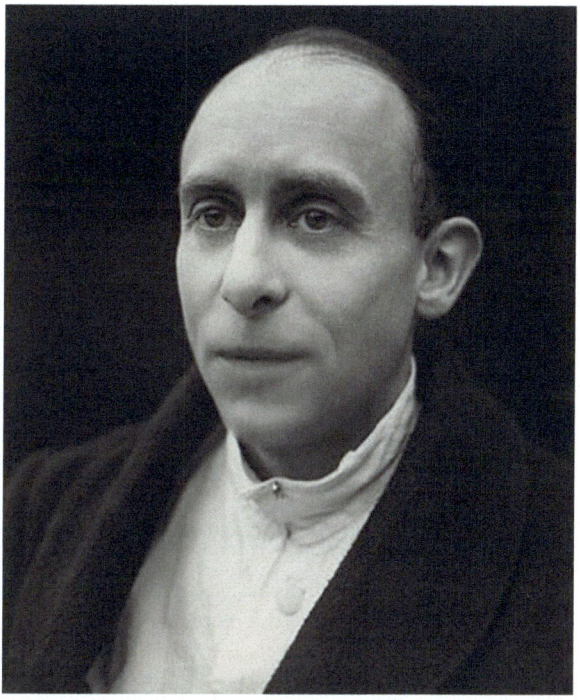

But the pivotal figure, the surgeon who seemed to bring together the accomplishments of his forbearers into a cohesive system of anatomic liver surgery, was Jacques Hepp (1905–1995) (Fig. 10.1). Jacques was the son of *Professeur* Maurice Hepp, who, in the early 1900s, developed techniques for the isolation of gastric juice in the pig model in his elaborate laboratories at Versailles, just outside of Paris. He identified a substance in gastric juice that, when injected into the stomachs of living dogs, produced a flow of liquid seemingly weeping from the stomach lining. He named this substance "Stimuline"—very likely the forerunner of the hormone, gastrin—a stimulator of the so-called "pneumogastric nerve." In fact, this concoction was bottled and marketed as "Hepptine," as a tonic for the relief of dyspepsia in the United States. While the younger Hepp was largely ignored by his socialite father, his mother was doting and attentive. She cherished her son, striving to smother him with the attention deprived by his aloof father. Jacques was sent to the prestigious *Lycée Hoche* in Versailles, a school known for its pipeline into some of the most exclusive of graduate schools. It was here that Jacques met Raymond Aron, with whom he would develop a lifelong connection both in friendship and the humanistic decency espoused by this philosopher comrade.[7] Despite the intense

---

[7] Raymond Aron (1905–1983) was a moderate voice in France's post-World War II political theater, denouncing Marxism as the opium of the intellectuals and promoting capitalism as part of a mixed economy of less radical leanings.

competitiveness of his secondary education, Jacques excelled, and, for a time, entertained a literary career, pursuits quite different from those of his busy father. However, with the encouragement, maybe even pressure, from his father, Jacques acquiesced to a path into medicine. He was equally brilliant in that quest graduating with distinction and gaining internships under the most sought after "masters" of the era, including *Professeur* Gosset at the *Hôpital Salpêtrière*.

It was from him that the young Hepp was first exposed to the liver and may have ignited his interest in hepatobiliary conditions. In 1929, at the age of 24, Hepp married Mademoiselle Myriam Le Bargy, daughter of the famous French actor and film director Monsieur Charles Le Bargy in a sumptuous Paris ceremony. He would forever be part of that elite Parisian intellectual circle and even aid his wife in her literary efforts. Professionally, for a more junior mentor, Hepp was drawn to Jean Charrier, one of Gosset's more trusted assistants and contributing author of Gosset's massive surgical text *Techniques Chirurgicales* published in 1936. Charrier would become an important mentor and friend. A skillful surgeon in his own right, Charrier would captivate his students with the rigor and thoroughness of his operative technique, described by one of his pupils, Jean Loygue, as simply "beautiful."

In 1938, now 33, Hepp was promoted to *chirurgien des hôpitaux*, the loose equivalent of an American chief resident, within the public hospital system, and was appointed as first assistant to the renowned André Bergeret. Hepp became Bergeret's man at the *Hopital Saint-Antoine*. It was likely Bergeret who nurtured that spark of interest in biliary conditions and, no doubt, supplied abundant clinical material for the young Hepp. On one occasion he recalled seeing Bergeret perform a pancreaticoduodenectomy in 1947, one of the first in France, "*de façon étourdissante et originale*" ("in a stunning and original manner") without, according to Hepp, copying other surgical descriptions, probably meaning those from America where the operation had gained some notoriety at the hands of Alan Whipple [11]. Maurice Mercadier, a young intern at the time, worked with both Bergeret and Hepp. While he described Bergeret as grand and fearless, an imposing figure—no doubt with some of the "brutish" qualities of his mentor, Hartmann, Hepp was described by Mercadier as "*délicat*" and reserved, courteous and pleasant, warm and humble. Hepp shared some of the values of his friend, Raymond Aron, "be honest everywhere, particularly at home," Aron had once said. Hepp took that to heart, honest to a fault, not afraid to point out inadequacies of France's public hospital system, the *Assistance Publique Hôpitaux*, its organization, hospital services, limitations on research, and experimental surgery, yet, at the same time, deferential and respectful. And in the operating room he was delicate as well, "elegant" as Mercadier described. He stressed complete exposure, careful exploration of the operative site, thorough and meticulous repair to the finest detail, and rigorous hemostasis. Mercadier was taken by the introspective young surgeon. "It was at *Saint-Antoine* that I met my spiritual father" he would later say [12].

Hepp's place of practice, the *Hôpital Saint-Antoine* had a rich and storied past in context of Parisian health care. It had been a former abbey, housing feminine penitents under the *règle de Cîteaux* (Order of Cisterciens), the *abbaye Saint-Antoine-des-Champs*, where it remained, under royal protection for the next few several centuries. With the tragic fire of the *Hôtel-Dieu* in 1772, the abbey was enlarged to create more space for reception of patients and the entire abbey was abolished with the Revolution in 1791, installing a new hospital to serve the population of east Paris, the *faubourg* Saint-Antoine. Seventy-two beds were built, all contained in two large ward-rooms, one for men and the other for females. But funds soon evaporated and the facility lapsed into disrepair, rubble strewn about and hygiene at a low level. Death rates soared from the deplorable conditions and incompetent staff. The Sisters of Saint Martha took over the hospital in 1811 and drastically improved conditions until mortality rates were within reason. As part of the public hospital system of Paris, Saint-Antoine slowly developed a reputable faculty, an active research effort, and notable physicians such as *Professeur* Hepp, specializing in digestive diseases and hematology. Modernized in the 1950s the hospital was chosen as headquarters of the *Centre Hospitalier Universitaire* of Paris, swelling to contain over 1000 beds.

At *Saint-Antoine*, under the leadership of Bergeret, Hepp would collaborate with a physician named Jacques Caroli (1902–1979). Caroli, while not a surgeon, had taken an interest in laying bare the anatomy of the biliary tract and investigating biliary pathology. He expanded the work of his mentor, the great Paul Carnot (1869–1957), *Professeur* of therapeutic medicine and *médecin des hôpitaux de Paris*, who began a study of the biliary system in patients with external biliary fistulas through the use of radiopaque contrast media. He was also aware of the work done by the Argentinian surgeon Pablo Luis Mirizzi (1893–1964) who, on June 18, 1931, performed the first operative cholangiogram, visualizing radiographically the intra- and extrahepatic biliary system using the contrast medium Lipiodol [13]. With the support and vast referral practice of the great Bergeret, Caroli began to accumulate an experience in contrast visualization of the biliary system even accompanied by manometric determinations, a technique he called *radiomanometre*. This was first employed in 1945 at the *Hôpital Saint-Antoine* on Bergeret's service, with Hepp as the surgeon. Caroli was enamored with his new device. His passion was such that he was invariably in the operating room, participating in the performance of his new "cholangiography" and measuring biliary pressures, exchanging information with the operating surgeon, often himself gowned and gloved. In fact, he developed a device for the operating room dubbed the "sarcophagus" by his colleagues. It was a large rectangular trunk in which could be placed the radiologist. A window would afford a view of the patient. An overhead X-ray tube could then slide over the patient and films taken, developed in an adjacent room, and read immediately in the operating room. Despite the criticisms of some that the surgeon was relegated to the role of a technician in all this, Jacques Hepp, for one, felt Caroli's technology, interest, and presence in the operating room was an example of remarkable ingenuity and teamwork. For liver surgery this was the dawn of multidisciplinary care [14].

But it was a partnership with his contemporary Claude Couinaud that would launch Hepp's notoriety and punctuate his genius. Hepp was intrigued with the biliary system, heretofore largely unchartered territory. His clinical investigations led to a number of publications, offering surgical options for hepaticolithiasis and techniques of utilizing the gastrointestinal tract for biliary reconstruction. Hepp was intrigued by Couinaud's description of the segmental anatomy of the liver, the configuration of the biliary tree, and the enveloping sheath of Glisson. By releasing—some called the maneuver "dropping" —the so-called "hilar plate" of Couinaud, Hepp could reach and expose the lengthy left hepatic duct. Here a broad anastomosis to jejunum could be fashioned, producing relief of hilar strictures—the now famous Hepp-Couinaud hepatico-jejunostomy [15]. Along with another confrere, surgeon Pierre Hautefeuille, Hepp, incorporating cholangiographic techniques of Caroli, thus radiographically visualizing intrahepatic bile ducts to identify precise ways to reconstruct the short, early branchings of right-sided biliary radicles. His methods were novel. Now, almost any biliary radical could be accessible [16].

In the background in those exciting years was a polite, slight of build surgical trainee by the name of Henri Bismuth. Bismuth was born in the North African French colony of Tunisia in 1934 of Jewish heritage and attended the prestigious *Lycée Carnot* in Tunis. His father, Joseph, was an inspector for the French *Postes, Télégraphes et Téléphones* (PTT)—the French postal service. Under protection by the Italian occupiers during World War II, the family had escaped the ethnic purges of the Nazis, and finally were liberated by the Allies in 1943. After medical school in Paris, Henri, *le fils*, had begun his surgical training in 1956 in the public hospital system, and identified Jacques Hepp early on as a mentor. The field of liver and biliary surgery was new, exciting, and fertile ground for pioneers like his teacher *Professeur* Hepp. By that time Hepp had moved to the *Hôpital Bichat* near Neuilly-sur-Seine. With his reputation the place had become a magnet for young "digestive" surgeons, flourishing under Hepp's fatherly guidance. Hepp's service, according to Jean Moreaux, Hepp's primary assistant at *Bichat*, was small—the "boss," one assistant (at the time usually Moreaux), three interns, and a foreign resident. With such an intimate gathering and with Hepp's paternal influence the whole experience seemed a close-knit family affair. Working with Moreaux, Hepp had argued in favor of extensive hepatic resections for primary liver cancers, even after the American Thomas Starzl had introduced hepatic transplantation [17]. As for young Bismuth, following formal surgical training, he, too, focused on the liver and biliary system— by that time Hepp's interest were primarily biliary—and Hepp was his man. For Bismuth Hepp would become more than a mentor, almost a father figure. Jacques Hepp, the introspective, polite aristocrate, the gifted surgeon would draw from the retiscent Bismuth a brilliance of his own, and watch a genius emerge.

Particularly challenging were problems encountered with end-stage liver disease and portal hypertension—the onerous catastrophes of bleeding esophageal varices. Bismuth had performed a number of portocaval anastomoses in rats and had been working with Hepp to perfect arterioportography as a way to visualize the portal system. His efforts eventually led to splenorenal shunts in humans with cirrhosis in the 1960s. Pupil accompanied master, assisting at his operations, more or less his "fellow." It was there in 1964 that Bismuth met the acquaintance of the Vietnamese surgeon Ton That Tung, who was visiting the Bichat Hospital in Neuilly with two of his colleagues. Tung later commented on their meeting, describing Bismuth as a "very sympathetic man" and with whom he would develop a lifelong friendship. Bismuth, in turn, was impressed with Tung and would adopt some of his techniques in liver resection, eventually ascribing his stepwise ritual of liver resection— "*réglée*" in the French—to the intense Vietnamese. *Réglée* would come to mean a predictable process of hepatectomy: first, isolating and controlling blood supply and biliary drainage, then methodically separating parenchyma along segmental boundaries as Couinaud had defined them (Bismuth had always considered Couinaud the quintessential anatomist). The end result was a safe and relatively bloodless operation.[8] So it would be Bismuth who lent clinical respectability to Couinaud's anatomic studies. Based on Couinaud's meticulous anatomic work Bismuth would provide a wealth of experience in segmental hepatic resection. By 1982, 22 of these segmentectomies had been performed, virtually all of Couinaud's segments successfully expunged. And in each case Bismuth carefully and thoroughly described his operative approach, even bringing into play techniques of Ton That Tung that he had incorporated. Bismuth's brilliance was in combining disciplines, providing a sound anatomic basis for hepatic resection, advancing surgical capabilities and care of patients.

[M]ajor and minor hepatic segmentectomies "*réglées*" are one of the best illustrations of the anatomical surgery of the liver. They are not techniques "*de facilité*" [easy] which can be chosen for a rapid and expeditious surgery [18].

Still, Bismuth was distracted by the numbers of patients suffering from biliary cirrhosis—those patients of Hepp who, after years of surgical management, inexorably developed the portal fibrosis and regenerative nodules characteristic of end-stage reaction to chronic biliary obstruction. In the 1960s, nothing short of total liver replacement would reverse the down-hill spiral. He began paying attention to the American surgeon Thomas Starzl and his ground-breaking work in human liver transplantation.

Bismuth had a vison for liver and biliary surgery. His intent was a center of excellence, one devoted only to those diseases and conditions. It was not a new idea. Hospitals around Paris had, for years, focused on select diseases. It was only when Bismuth was reappointed to a position at the *Hôpital Paul Brousse* that his idea crystallized. *Hôpital Paul Brousse*, named after the French physician, socialist, and reformist who died in 1912, began service in the sleepy Paris suburb of Villejuif (Val-de-Marne) in 1913. As the name implied, the town contained a large Jewish population. The vintage stone structure built was first designed to serve the elderly and those terminally ill—as much a free-standing hospice as anything else. By 1919, the first oncology service in France opened, morphing into the Gustave Roussy Cancer Institute in 1942. In 1961, *Paul Brousse* became part of the *Assistance Publique—Hôpitaux de Paris* but continued its mission as a center of gerontology and oncology. In 1964, the hospital hosted one of the first French *Institut national de la santé et de la recherché medical* (Institute of Health and Medical Research—INSERM), directed by André Monsaingeon (1912–1997). *Professeur* Monsaingeon

---

[8] Daniel Azoulay, personal communication with Henri Bismuth, January, 2016.

was head of surgery at *Paul Brousse*, appointed in 1947, and had spent a year at the Massachusetts General Hospital with Dr. Francis Moore as a Rockefeller Fellow in burns [19].[9] On his return to Paris Monsaingeon attempted to model INSERM after the American National Institutes of Health and began a research program at *Paul Brousse* for burns and experimental surgery. At that time *Paul Brousse* was—in vernacular terms—little more than a hospice whose residents were either elderly or hopelessly ill. The modernization program instituted by *Professeur* Monsaingeon would lift surgical services to a more respected level and provide solid clinical footing and respectability for the former hospice. One of his chief accomplishments, though, was the recruitment of Henri Bismuth to *Paul Brousse*. By 1970, Bismuth had ascended the academic ladder and attained the rank of *Chirurgien des hôpitaux de Paris* and *Professeur*. His next assignment was at the *Hôpital Paul Brousse*. The two would change the face of liver surgery in Paris.

References

1. Weisz G (2001) Reconstructing Paris medicine. Bull Hist Med 75:105–119
2. Weisz G (2003) The emergence of medical specialization in the nineteenth century. Bull Hist Med 77:536–574
3. Weisz G (1994) Mapping medical specialization in Paris in the nineteenth and twentieth centuries. Social Hist Med 7:177–211
4. Guivarc'h M (2005) La Réforme Farabeuf de l'Enseignement Pratique de l'Anatomie et de la Médecine Opératoire: Dix Ans Rue Vaquelin 1877-1886. Hist Sci Med 34:45–57
5. Merola L (1919) Anatomia del Peritoneo Hepatico. An Fac de Med, Montevideo 4:61–68
6. Merola L (1920) Manera de abordar la cara superior del hígado: Incisión toraco-abdominal. Anales de la Universidad (Uruguay) 108:108–111
7. Caprio G (1931) Un Caso de Extirpación del Lóbulo Izquierdo del Hígado. Bol Soc Cir Urug 2:159–163
8. Martinez LR (2019) Caprio and Merola: Latin American contribution to the development of liver surgery. Dig Surg 36:124–128
9. Means TA (1857) Parisian hospitals–their more striking features and advantages. Atlanta Med Surg J 3:1–14
10. Steudler F (1973) Hôpital, Profession Médicale et Politique Hospitalière. Rev Fr Sociol 14:13–40
11. Edelmann G (1977) André Bergeret 1884-1969. Chirurgie 103:11–22
12. Moreaux J (2003) Éloge de Maurice Mercadier. Bull Acad Natle Med 187:1041–1050
13. Mirizzi PZ (1932) La Colangiograffea Durante las Operacione de les Vias Biliares. Bol y trab de la Soc de cir de Buenos Aires 16:1133–1161
14. Caroli JH (1955) Sur les Indications de l'Angiocholegraphi Intra-Hépatique Percutanée et des Anastomoses Biliaires Intra-Hépatique. Rev Med Chir Mal Foie 30:39–56
15. Hepp J, Couinaud C (1956) L'Abord et l'Utilisation de Canal Hépatique Gauche dans les Réparations de la Voie Biliare Principale. Presse Med 64:947–948

---

[9]André Monsaingeon wrote an interesting article in *Presse Medicale* about his experiences in Boston in 1966 and the advances in American surgery including transplantation, sepsis, and shock, those notable areas where Dr. Moore had been so vigorously involved [20].

16. Hepp JP et al (1966) Les Lésions Concernant la Convergence en Chirurgie Biliaire Réparatrice. Ann Chir 20:382–411
17. Mercadier M (1997) Éloge de Jacques Hepp (1905-1995). Bull Acad Natle Med 181:9–16
18. Bismuth HH et al (1982) Major and minor Segmentectomies "Réglées" in liver surgery. World J Surg 6:10–24
19. Francis D, Moore MD (1995) A miracle and a privilege: recounting a half century of surgical advance. Joseph Henry Press, Boston
20. Monsaingeon A (1966) C d'œil sur la vie chirurgicale à Boston. Presse Med 74:2501–2506

Chapter 11
Bach, Beethoven, and Brahms

They would be called the Bach, Beethoven, and Brahms of liver surgery—Henri Bismuth, Stig Bengmark, and Leslie Blumgart—virtuosos in the surgical symphony of liver diseases. Each would make contributions in liver resection which would thrust the field into the modern era. Bismuth with his concepts of multidisciplinary care, Bengmark with his efforts to unite the liver communities, and Leslie Blumgart, who would expand liver resection to numbers of patients once considered hopelessly incurable.

In Paris Henri Bismuth pursued his dream: to create a center for liver and biliary surgery. It was there, in 1974, that he performed the first liver transplant in France, one of only three such programs at that time in continental Europe. By 1977 he had become Chief of the Surgery Service at *Paul Brousse* and shortly assembled a multidisciplinary team of specialists—including intensivists, hepatologists, radiologists, and "endoscopists"—all under his control, to focus on diseases of the liver and biliary system. In 1993, his *Centre Hépato-biliare*, adjacent to the *Hôpital Paul Brousse*, opened—a multilevel all-inclusive setting for patients to receive specialty care, including liver transplantation. Bismuth and his team soon achieved international preeminence in liver surgery. "My hepatobiliary center in Paris is a model of this [holistic care] ... It is no more the department of surgery, but the department of liver diseases, where all specialists work together," he told an interviewer in 2013 [1, 2]. Like his forebearers Bismuth would train a new generation of hepatic surgeons, instructing in that quiet, repetitive manner from which he had learned. One of his pupils, Denis Castaing would later say:

> The apprenticeship I had undergone under his [Bismuth's] tutelage was truly Socratic, limned in the logic and comportment of a master teacher, with learning by observation, by imitation, and by correction ... I learned everything by listening to him, watching him, and assisting him [3].

It was the French method. The high volume of liver cases seen at his *Centre Hépato-biliare* provided the regulated, repetition so necessary for smooth, efficient

T. S. Helling, D. Azoulay, *Historical Foundations of Liver Surgery*,
https://doi.org/10.1007/978-3-030-47095-1_11

operations. Without actually being led through these procedures Bismuth's students, after so many opportunities, would know, almost instinctively, the steps, the movements, the roles of surgeon and assistant at the operating table day after day that were vital to the success of complex liver operations. It was as if the air and all human forms stilled only to move at the direction of the maestro Bismuth. With practiced delicacy each motion and counter-motion were completed as if incessantly rehearsed and now second nature such as one knows the rhythms of breathing or the pivoting dalliances of a tango or the swift and intricate ties of fine suture. Words were no longer necessary—only expectations. Castaing was aware of that when asked to do a portocaval shunt on his own. Flawless. "At that moment," he said, "I could truly measure the remarkable teaching I had received." [3].

To Padua to learn from the hands of the Italian Pettinari that the young surgeon Stig Bengmark was sent. His mentor Professor Ragnar Romanus at the University of Gothenborg in 1961 had hopes of developing a first-class liver program, and the inquisitive Bengmark seemed tailored to the task. Romanus instructed Bengmark to see one liver resection before trying it himself. With money from the Volvo car manufacturer (loosely related to automotive trauma) he spent over a month waiting for Pettinari to perform just one liver resection, a limited left lobectomy (left segmentectomy). "A fantastic show," Bengmark later remembered and euphemistically added "[n]ow there should be no obstacles to our starting to build a section of hepatic surgery in Lund" [4]. Back to Gothenborg and the start of his own program, all questions answered in that one brief case—"one and done" so the saying goes.[1] Despite the inactivity, Bengmark hardly minded the respite from clinical duties, and seemed quite certain he was prepared to begin his journey into liver surgery. More than anything, it seemed, he reveled in the Italian *dolce vita*. He would later reminisce: "My young wife and I spent some of the most wonderful times of our lives in Padua, enjoying the splendid climate in late spring and the Italian lifestyle." [4].

Stig Bengmark was born in Ostervala, Sweden, in 1929. He had been drawn to the physiology of experimental liver regeneration while working on his PhD at Lund University and continued his efforts after moving to Gothenborg where he set up his first research laboratory in 1959. Fascinated by early work in liver surgery, he was keen on carrying his experimental work to the bedside, applying hepatic resection to tumorous conditions, and involving a clinical team of collaborators: Olle Almersjo, Lennart Engevik, and Larsolof Hafstrom. In short order they began their clinical work, producing a noteworthy publication on major hepatic resections by 1966 [5]. Not satisfied merely with developing a large clinical practice, Bengmark, the intellectual, focused on derangements initiated by resection and the ability of the liver to compensate—the "fantastic capacity" to regenerate as he called it—that permitted surgeons to remove large portions. He soon became an authority in the field, producing a number of clinical and experimental papers on factors promoting

---

[1] It is not unusual for visiting surgeons to glean much of what is needed for a new operative procedure from just one exposure. "See one, do one, teach one" has some historic basis.

and inhibiting hepatic renewal.[2] But like many surgeons of the era, Bengmark would remain the total surgeon with a broad range of interests from nutrition to bacterial translocation to surgical emergencies. In 1970, Bengmark was chosen to replace the legendary Phillip Sandblom as head of the Department of Surgery at Lund University and to continue his pioneering work. The distinguished Professor Sandblom (1903–2001) had initiated programs in experimental surgery and chronic liver disease and served as the Chair of Surgery and then Vice-Chancellor of the University. As with many developing liver centers, Sandblom had become involved in portal hypertension surgery and had amassed an enviable experience of portocaval shunts for acute variceal bleeding, reducing postoperative mortality to close to 10% [7].[3] However, it would be his successor, Stig Bengmark, who would accelerate the growing interest in liver resection for metastatic cancer, adding immensely to the clinical material available for liver surgeons. But Bengmark well appreciated his roots and had an undying respect for his mentor and predecessor, Sandblom. "The opportunity to build an HPB centre [sic] on the foundations laid by Professor Sandblom was exciting" [4]. An inveterate researcher, Bengmark commented "My burning interest in research and the conditions offered [at Lund] made it natural to focus on experimental research and communication between scientists" [4]. His intent was to develop a network of surgeons committed to hepatic surgery so that sharing of information would advance the field far faster than one clinician could do. Stig Bengmark would forge a new association of like-minded surgeons, propelling liver and biliary surgery from individual heroic efforts in clinical and research centers scattered across Europe to a dynamic field, fueled by a cooperative exchange of ideas and information. Bengmark was particularly interested in drawing his Asian colleagues into the fold. He well understood the talent that awaited exposure to the international community but also realized that lack of funding, language barriers, and even lack of education on how to write a "westernized" abstract or manuscript retarded their involvement. For that reason, Bengmark was instrumental in setting up various educational programs culminating in the International World Congress on HPB surgery (now called the International Hepato-Pancreato-Biliary Association) in 1986.

Leslie Blumgart was born in Johannesburg, South Africa, in 1931. He attended the University of Witwatersrand in Johannesburg, receiving his dental degree in 1954. Blumgart then embarked on a dental practice for 5 years in the coastal town of Durban, South Africa. Dissatisfied with the inhumanity of apartheid and longing for a career in medicine, he traveled to England, entering medical school at the University of Sheffield and graduating in 1962. Then it was to the Royal Hospital of

---

[2] By 1970 he was a recognized international figure in hepatic regeneration and wrote the chapter on regeneration in George T. Pack and Abdol H. Islami's text [6].

[3] To Phillip Sandblom would be attributed the term "hemobilia" first described by him in 1948. He later, in 1970, would coin the term "hemosuccus pancreaticus," bleeding into the pancreatic duct and into the gastrointestinal tract through the sphincter of Oddi. In addition Sandblom and his wife, Grace, were inveterate patrons of the arts, collecting a number of masterpieces in their lavish home. A "citizen of the world," he was called (see [8]).

Sheffield, working under the distinguished Sir Andrew Watt Kay when he was chair of surgery. Blumgart completed his tenure as registrar at Sheffield in 1970, having spent 2 years as a research fellow in addition to his clinical duties. Like many "general surgeons" at the time, his work spanned a spectrum of surgical diseases, publishing on subjects from gastric freezing (once in vogue for ulcer disease) to breast cancer to blunt abdominal trauma. Yet throughout was a deepening curiosity with biliary and hepatic physiology and regeneration that would become his trademark in later years. In fact, at Nottingham General Hospital near Sheffield, in 1967, Blumgart participated in his first hepatic resection with colleague Michael Baum. Blumgart's first faculty appointment was at the Cardiff Royal Infirmary in 1970, and in 1972 he was named the St. Mungo Professor of Surgery at the Glasgow Royal Infirmary. It was in Cardiff that he developed his interest in liver surgery, frustrated by attempts to salvage victims of massive liver trauma. It was mostly self-education, his only stimulus a burning desire to salvage these moribund patients. Two cases in particular seemed unnecessarily tragic, a 16-year-old boy and a 21-year-old man, both of whom bled to death from their liver injuries treated by suturing and packing. "Experience in these two cases convinced us of the need to adopt a more aggressive surgical approach, and formal resection of the liver was performed … in the four subsequent cases of similar extensive injury." In the five cases of hepatectomy after trauma that he then reported, two died of their associated injuries. All apparently survived the rather formidable undertaking of hepatectomy in the face of hemorrhagic shock. All had extensive, stellate-type wounds of the right liver. All but one patient required 18 units or more of blood.

Blumgart had prepared. He had intensely studied the literature and operative methods of established liver surgeons. Even though these were emergency cases, his technique was painstaking, as if he and his colleagues were embarking on an elective, controlled, "*reglee*" type of resection—isolation, ligation, and division of vascular pedicles at the hilum, mobilization of the right liver off the diaphragm and bare area, and even ligation of the right hepatic vein. He modeled his method after the anatomic studies of Lloyd-Davies and Angell from Saint Mark's Hospital, London, published in 1957 [9] and after the approach of Quattlebaum and Quattlebaum [10]. Lloyd-Davies went into great detail to explain his operative rationale, based on careful anatomic dissection of livers in the "postmortem" room. His first reported right lobectomy "was based entirely on these experiences," he penned.

Lloyd-Davies had placed his patient in a "half-left lateral" position and performed a wide incision extending from thoracic cavity, across the costal margin and into the abdomen. The diaphragm was divided down to the inferior vena cava foramen, widely exposing the liver and, in fact, facilitating exposure in that the liver literally fell into the chest cavity, thus enhancing the view of the portal fissure. Then the hilum was addressed, isolating the hepatic artery, right hepatic duct, and right branch of the portal vein. Only then was the right (or, subsequently, the left) lobe mobilized, dividing the right or left triangular ligament and gaining access (on the right) to the bare area of the liver and retrohepatic vena cava. He tilted the patient to the left "to allow the liver to fall to that side"—almost in a left lateral position. The "short" hepatic veins were ligated and divided. Here Lloyd-Davies pointed out the tongue of liver and ligamentous tissue later termed the hepato-caval ligament hiding the right hepatic vein and how this must be divided to gain access to the hepatic vein. "It is often quite adherent and needs careful dissection to avoid injury to the great veins," he cautioned.[4] The hepatic vein was then encircled, ligated, and divided. "This was the most precarious part of the operation," he recounted, "but its safe accomplishment made the operation feasible." The patient was then turned to a neutral position, the liver once again fell back into the chest, and the porta hepatis exposed. Only then were the right hepatic artery, the right hepatic duct, and the right branch of the portal vein ligated and divided. Once accomplished, the gallbladder was removed, and the liver parenchyma was divided along the oblique plane of Couinaud, using the scalpel, "only a few small vessels being encountered which could be seized with forceps and tied," he reported (based on his one case report).[5] Parenchymal control was obtained with catgut sutures, eventually transfixing the raw liver surface for hemostasis. While substantial, blood loss was probably less due to the hypovolemic state of these patients, an observation that did not escape the young Blumgart, fostering a practice of lowering central venous pressure even in elective cases.

Blumgart's success prompted a policy at the Royal Cardiff Infirmary of routine hepatic resection in the case of "pulped" liver. "We now advocate liver resection for extensive liver lacerations," was his conclusion [11]. And the fire had been lit. Success in these critically injured patients would provide a solid springboard for less urgent operations on no less seriously ill patients riddled with cancer. Familiar with prior ligation of structures in the porta hepatis, Blumgart would also be heavily influenced by the intraparenchymal approach described by Professor Bernard Launois in Rennes, France, the same approach advocated by the Vietnamese sur-geon Tôn Thất Tùng, in which hilar control, other than clamping *en masse, a la* James Pringle, is forsaken in favor of pedicle exposure *inside* the liver substance, providing a clearer picture of segmental liver anatomy [12]:

> The technique has many advantages: being rapid and achievable with little blood loss and allowing not only control of bleeding and biliary leakage, but … allowing definition of the parenchymal territory supplied by those pedicles …

---

[4] It was a unique observation and, indeed, true. Surprisingly, this important step was seldom men-tioned by other anatomists and surgeons in describing approaches to right hepatic "lobectomy." Lloyd-Davies also provided a series of startlingly accurate anatomic drawings, quite pertinent for defining surgical anatomy of the liver.

[5] The Quattlebaums disagreed here. "Division of the liver with a sharp instrument results in profuse hemorrhage which is difficult to control … Therefore the section is made … with a blunt instru-ment, such as the handle of a knife, a closed scissors, or small clamp," they felt [10, p. 649]. Lloyd-Davies' case may have fortuitously had a clean division of right and left livers, a situation recognized—and enjoyed—only too infrequently by liver surgeons. Indeed it could be called the "sweet spot" of liver surgery.

The man largely responsible for Blumgart's early successes in liver resection was Oswald Vaughn Lloyd-Davies (1905–1987). Lloyd-Davies was born at Cheriton, Kent, just across the channel from Calais. He was the son of Reverend Samuel Lloyd-Davies, a Welsh congregational minister. He received his medical education at Middlesex Hospital in London, graduating in 1930. While still a student he was an anatomy tutor and prosector. Within 6 years of graduation he was appointed to the surgical staff at Saint Mark's Hospital at the age of 30. His interest lay in rectal surgery, particularly patients with rectal cancer. A major achievement was his perfection of the lithotomy-Trendelenburg position for simultaneous abdominal and perineal resection of rectal tumors. Simultaneously, Lloyd-Davies also refined techniques for low anastomoses of colon to rectum, thus sparing sphincters and avoiding permanent colostomies. This was to earn him the reputation as a founding fathers of colon and rectal surgery.[6] His rather oblique interest in liver surgery was typical of surgeons of the era, his particular fascination the result of metastases to the liver from colon and rectum. Lloyd-Davies was described as a modest and self-effacing gentleman who operated in a steady, meticulous manner. Aside from his painstaking technique of liver resection, described in 1957, he had already performed a topographical left lobectomy in 1947 for a metastatic deposit of rectal cancer ("not a particularly formidable task," he wrote) and simultaneously performed a proctectomy on the same patient for the primary lesion [13]. His major focus was colon and rectal surgery, however, and besides the various sphincter-preserving techniques, he also designed a number of instruments for these occasions [14].

It was in Scotland, too, that Blumgart, working in concert with the gastroenterologist Peter Cotton at Saint Thomas Hospital, London, began clinical use of the side-viewing fiberoptic duodenoscope in cannulating the ampulla of Vater, achieving visualization of the biliary and pancreatic ductal systems, the first surgeon to be involved in this dramatic diagnostic advancement [15]. His work in this area would result in a number of publications, establishing retrograde cholangiopancreatography as an essential adjunct to biliary and pancreatic surgery. Still Blumgart was not to be distracted from his primary pursuit of the intricacies of liver resection, its place in clinical surgery, and its necessary accompaniment, regeneration. Like Bengmark, Blumgart was intrigued by the remarkable ability of mammalian liver to initiate the rapid process of hyperplasia and hypertrophy that, in some animal models, occurred over a period of days. His curiosity in liver regeneration prompted visits to the American genius, Thomas Starzl, whose work on this subject in his Denver laboratories was uncovering promoters of this phenomenon carried in portal blood flow. Like Starzl, Blumgart performed manipulations of rat and dog liver including alterations of portal blood flow and their effects on liver regeneration.

In the meantime, Blumgart would turn his attention from liver trauma to liver tumors. In particular, patients such as those Lloyd-Davies had reported with colon or rectal cancer metastases led him to believe that resection of such liver deposits

---

[6] From: "Oswald Vaughn Lloyd-Davies, Obituary", *Lancet*, (1987) 2:465 (no author)

might afford a cure. But it was Bengmark who early on followed the natural history of patients with metastatic colon and rectal cancer. Bengmark was impressed by the dire fate of those patients, recounting that of the 38 in his sample size, none were alive 2 years later. He was led to the conclusion that "hepatic metastases constitute an important factor in the survival of patients" [16]. Yet it was Blumgart who would suggest, several years later, that some of these patients could survive for years, if not indefinitely, if those metastatic lesions could be removed. Of 113 patients so afflicted those with solitary lesions—even a limited number of lesions—seemed to fare better, a few even surviving beyond 3 years [17]. He became a crusader for such events, insisting that surgical extirpation was an essential component of therapy. And Connecticut surgeon James Foster would prove it. Traveling around the country in his Volkswagen, the Hartford clinician and epidemiologist amassed a sizeable number of cases of liver resection for metastatic colon and rectal cancer, finding, in fact, that over one-fifth of patients were alive 5 years after their resections:

> Resection of metastases must remain a most controversial subject, but this collected data should give encouragement to the surgeon when he encounters localized and solitary metastatic disease of the liver [18].[7]

Such observations did not escape the attention of Blumgart. With the number of individuals developing colon and rectal cancer, one of the top three cancers worldwide, an enormous pool of patients was potentially available for liver resection. By Blumgart's calculations, over one-third of these patients would develop liver metastases, many of whom could be candidates for resection. Rather than the occasional forays by individual surgeons into the liver for spectacular resections, hepatic surgery now could be made available to a wider spectrum of patients, many of whom suffered from neoplastic diseases formerly considered incurable.

What revolutionized oncologic surgery on the liver was the introduction of imaging modalities capable of penetrating the human frame to give a pictorial display of intra-abdominal organs, particularly liver substance. Development of computerized axial tomography (CT scanning) was, in the words of Geoffrey Rubin:

> [A] triumph of ingenuity in engineering and applied physics. Its unparalleled evolution over the past 40 years is a testament to the power of academic and industry collaboration across many disciplines in medicine, science, and engineering [20].

Developed by electrical engineer Sir Godfrey Hounsfield and physicist Allan Cormack in 1971,[8] the whole-body CT scanner entered medical practice in 1975. Over the next quarter century CT scanners increased in complexity and resolution

---

[7] Foster became the first full-time surgery director at the Hartford Hospital in 1968. His interests gradually shifted from general surgery (and renal transplantation) to liver tumors. His compendium of liver neoplasms, the culmination of his cross-country travels, written with colleague Martin Berman, became a landmark reference source, popular still, decades after its publication [19].

[8] For which they jointly received the Nobel Prize in Physiology or Medicine in 1979. For a brief biography of Hounsfield see [21].

allowing for unbelievably accurate depiction of visceral anatomy and unprecedented views of the human liver, even in three-dimension. Suddenly, physical examination took a back seat to radiographic intervention and routine scanning of asymptomatic individuals and gave opportunities for earlier, curative extirpation of primary or secondary hepatic cancers. Further refinements of imaging occurred with the introduction of magnetic resonance imaging (MRI) in 1977 by physician and mathematician Raymond Damadian. The MRI, as further refined by the American physicist William Edelstein, allowed unique views of abdominal organs, leading Frank Doyle and his colleagues to help establish an independent but complimentary role for MRI in imaging of the liver by 1982 [22, 23]. Combined with intraoperative B-mode real-time ultrasonography of the liver as developed by Makuuchi of Japan in the late 1970s hepatic imagery became as sensitive as postmortem dissections (if not more so) and assumed an integral role in determining the extent and distribution of liver lesions (see the review by [24]).

References

1. He VJ (2013) Professor Henri Bismuth: the past, present, and future of hepatobiliary surgery. Hepatobiliary Surg Nutr 2:236–238
2. Bismuth H (1999) The Centre Hépato-Biliaire, Villejuif, France. HPB 1:125–126
3. Castaing D (2016) Presidential address of professor Denis Castaing. J Visc Surg 153:243–247
4. Bengmark S (2002) The early days of HPB: a personal reminiscence. HPB 4:117–121
5. Engevik LA et al (1966) Hemihepatectomy in man. Acta Chir Scand Suppl 357:239–243
6. Bengmark S (1970) Liver regeneration. In: Pack GT (ed) Tumors of the liver. Springer-Verlag, New York, pp 187–212
7. Ekman CA, Sandblom P (1964) Shunt operation in acute bleeding from esophageal varices. Ann Surg 160:531–539
8. Ihse I (2001) Philip Sandblom; surgeon, scientist, humanist and citizen of the world. HPB 3:219–220
9. Lloyd-Davies OV, Angell JC (1957) Right hepatic lobectomy: operative technique, some anatomical points, and an account of a case. Br J Surg 45:113–117
10. Quattlebaum JK, Quattlebaum JK Jr (1959) Technique of hepatic lobectomy. Ann Surg 149:648–651
11. Blumgart LH, Vajrabukka T (1972) Injuries to the liver: analysis of 20 cases. Br Med J 1:158–164
12. Blumgart LH (2013) Forward. In: Launois B, Jamieson G (eds) The posterior intrahepatic approach in liver surgery. Springer, New York
13. Lloyd-Davies OV (1947) Carcinoma of the rectum with a single secondary in the liver, synchronous combined excision and left hepatectomy. Proc R Soc Med 40:875–876
14. Corman M (1989) Oswald Vaughan Lloyd-Davies 1905-1987. Dis Colon Rectum 32:172–175
15. Cotton PB et al (1972) Cannulation of papilla of vater via fiberduodenoscope. Lancet 1:53–58
16. Bengmark SH, Hafstrom L (1969) The natural history of primary and secondary malignant tumors of the liver. Cancer 23:198–202
17. Wood CB (1976) A retrospective study of the natural history of patients with liver metastases from colorectal cancer. Clin Oncol 2:285–288
18. Foster JH (1970) Survival after liver resection for cancer. Cancer 26:493–502
19. Foster JH, Berman MM (1977) Solid liver tumors. Saunders, Philadelphia

20. Rubin GD (2014) Computed tomography: revolutionizing the practice of medicine for 40 years. Radiology 273:S45–S74
21. Richmond C (2004) Sir Godfrey Hounsfield. BMJ 329:687
22. Doyle FH et al (1982) Nuclear magnetic resonance imaging of the liver: initial experience. Am J Roentgenol 138:193–200
23. Roth CG-D et al (2018) Contributions of magnetic resonance imaging to gastroenterological practice: MRIs for GIs. Dig Dis Sci 63:1102–1122
24. Makuuchi MT et al (1998) History of intraoperative ultrasound. Ultrasound Med Biol 24:1229–1242

Chapter 12
The Era of Transplantation

The slender, intense figure with a quick, disarming smile who prowled the halls of the gleaming Colorado General Hospital spanning Ninth Avenue in downtown Denver had been invited by the University of Colorado's Chair of Surgery, William Waddell to fill the Chief slot in surgery at the Denver Veterans Affairs Hospital. Doctor Waddell had recognized a streak of brilliance in the young Thomas Starzl, alerted to his accomplishments by his dear friend Ben Eiseman at the University of Kentucky by his dear friend Ben Eiseman at the University of Kentucky. Eiseman had developed a reputation as a talentscout for up-and-coming surgeons. Doctor Starzl had already become enthralled by the liver from his days in training at the University of Miami. He was fascinated by this "enormous and silent reddish-brown organ" that hid so many secrets of its purpose over the centuries and punished those foolish enough to venture into its deepest recesses [1]. In particular, one of the most challenging problems for surgeons of the era was the patient with cirrhosis who bled so copiously from large, fragile collateral veins engorged because of portal hypertension, the body's attempt to reroute blood around a scarred and obstinate liver. The enigmatic shrunken, blemished liver was the crux of the problem. Liver replacement was the inescapable solution. Little else was possible without major ramifications, few of them desirable. Such horrible hemorrhages in these desperately ill patients captivated the young Starzl and would launch his career in liver surgery (Fig. 12.1).

12.1 The Conundrum of Portal Hypertension

Leonardo da Vinci may well have been the first to recognize and write about the condition of portal hypertension. In one of his anatomic dissections he described enormous veins traveling to the liver, engorged and tortuous "like a snake," with the liver dried, and having the appearance of "frozen bran, in color and consistency." Da

Fig. 12.1 Thomas Starzl
(1926–2017) from
University of Pittsburgh
Medical Center

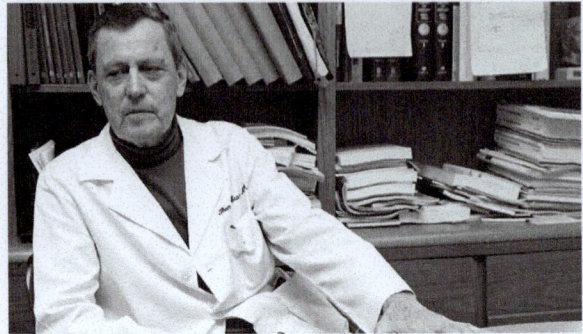

Vinci apparently thought that the mesenteric vein engorgement had caused the liver
to shrink and not the opposite [2].

Scattered reports in the seventeenth-century literature alluded to disorders of the
liver that some have interpreted as early descriptions of cirrhosis. John Brown, a surgeon of the Saint Thomas Hospital in Southwark, London, reported on the liver of a
25-year-old soldier who fell ill with "distemper," and died following a paracentesis for
anasarca and voluminous ascites. At autopsy the liver was found to contain "glands"
of a yellowish "ichor" (an unpleasant smelling, watery discharge) like pustules. Could
this have represented cirrhosis? It would certainly be unusual for such a young, apparently vigorous individual to suddenly develop a cirrhotic liver, although certainly a
type of acute hepatitis was more likely [3]. More to the point in 1793 British physician
and pathologist Matthew Baillie (1761–1823) detailed "tubercles" of the liver, associated with "hard drinkers" that occupy "the whole mass of the liver ... placed very near
each other, and are of a rounded shape," giving an irregular appearance to the liver's
surface. On cut surface they appear brownish or yellowish [4].

In telling of the autopsy of a 47-year-old man who had suffered from ascites and
a *maladie organique du foie* (an organic liver disease) with ascites, the inventor of the
stethoscope and renowned pulmonary pathologist, René Théophile Hyacinthe
Laennec (1781–1826) noted that the liver was reduced to one-third of its ordinary
size and exhibited a "hilly and wrinkled surface that gave a yellowish hue." Cutting
the parenchyma he found a multitude of small, round and oval granules, again with a
tawny color. Instead of using the more common term *squirrhe* (from the Greek *skir-
ros*, meaning hard or fibrotic) he preferred the term *cirrhose*, from the Greek *kirrhos*,
meaning orange-yellow ("I think I should call it cirrhosis because of its color," he
wrote). Lannaec observed as well that the liver in this condition is one of the most
common causes of ascites [5]. While not popular in France, Laennec, in large part
because of the great Sir William Osler's endorsement, would forever be linked to
micronodular cirrhosis. Osler would call it the "atrophic cirrhosis of Laennec," and
characterize those livers as "greatly reduced" in size with "numerous granulations on
the surface." That yellowish hue was indeed Laennec's cirrhosis [6].[1]

---

[1] For a riveting discussion of Laennec and his cirrhosis, see [7].

By the mid-nineteenth century many believed that occlusion of the portal vein in cirrhosis was the cause rather than effect of the liver disease. However, experiments in 1856 by French surgeon Pierre-Cyprien Oré (1828–1891) on dogs demonstrated that occlusion of the portal vein, if sudden, was indeed fatal (perhaps by pooling of splanchnic blood) but if slowly occluded the animals might not die and later autopsy showed that, while the portal vein was a fibrous cord and the liver diminished in volume—but still making bile and glycogen—the splanchnic circulation had established venous collaterals with the systemic circulation, thus introducing the concept of porto-systemic shunting as a way to decompress a visceral venous circulation hampered by portal occlusion. And livers of those animals continued to produce bile and metabolize glycogen [8]. Oré's conclusion was that the hepatic artery was responsible for the production of bile and processing of "sugars" (implying portal blood was not vital to liver viability), a presumption criticized by the editors of the American *Atlanta Medical and Surgical Journal* in a fit of trans-Atlantic rivalry:

> Can it be possible that the distinguished medical savans [sic] of the French Academy, are ignorant of the fact, established by Kiernan and others that the capillary terminations of the hepatic artery end in venous capillaries which open into the adjacent subdivisions of the portal vein ...? [9][2]

Yet, something ominous happened with portal blood deprivation. From Geneva in 1877 Swiss physician B.F. Lautenbach described the behavior of animals whose portal vein had been ligated. "[T]he animal passes into a state resembling that following a fatal dose of one of the narcotics," he observed. His only explanation was that "the blood of an animal in whom the vena porta has been tied must therefore contain a violent poison which does not exist ... in the blood of normal animals." In other words, could the liver be responsible for elimination of this "poison" from the circulation? [11] Lautenbach's article was seen by an eccentric Russian experimentalist named Nicolai Eck (1849–1908). What humors were harbored in the liver (or detoxified therein) was still a matter of conjecture. Eck set about proving that, in fact, dog livers could withstand portal occlusion. He perfected an arduous technique of establishing a porto-cava fistulous communication of splanchnic blood, diverting the entirety from the dog's liver. Seven of eight dogs survived beyond the operation and died, apparently, of "peritonitis or strangulation of the intestines and omentum." One dog that survived for over 2 months ran away and was never seen again. While Eck performed the operation in hopes of relieving ascites, he determined that portal blood could be diverted "without any danger to the body" and was "a perfectly safe operation" [12]. Not so, felt Ivan Pavlov (1849–1936) who, along with his collaborators, tested Eck's fistula on 60 dogs, 20 of whom survived. These dogs exhibited bizarre behavior when fed meat products, culminating, many times, in stupor and death. Eck's fistula was not an innocuous operation [13].

Moreover, in 1909, George Whipple and John Sperry at Johns Hopkins demonstrated severe liver changes in two dogs undergoing Eck fistulas. Both dogs became

---

[2] Irish surgeon Francis Kiernan (1800–1874) described the lobular architecture of the liver in 1833 including central veins and portal triads [10].

noticeably weak and sick appearing. "[T]he establishment of an Eck fistula causes considerable central atrophy and fatty degeneration," they noted, specifying that these changes even preceded treatment of the dogs with chloroform [14].

In 1883, French anatomist Constant Sappey (1810–1896) more or less confirmed the findings of Oré describing collateral circulation in cases of obstruction of the portal vein by cirrhosis. These collaterals he found primarily in the suspensory ligaments of the liver (falciform ligament), shuttling blood from the splanchnic circulation to the systemic circulation via subdiaphragmatic veins (Sappey's superior vein) or to epigastric veins of the anterior abdomen (Sappey's inferior veins). This system essentially comprised a large "bypass" around the liver. Sappey concluded that when these existed in the presence of cirrhosis it was a favorable sign, "since it removes the fear of abdominal dropsy" (ascites) [15]. This led British surgeons David Drummond and Rutherford Morison in 1896 (and later the German Sape Talma in 1898 [16]) to devise an operation intended to foster development of additional collaterals through abrasion of parietal peritoneum and attachment of the omentum to the abraded surfaces. At least in one reported case this effectively terminated the patient's intractable ascites and represented the first attempt at porto-systemic shunting [17].

It was in this era of the Drummond-Morison-Talma omentopexy that the first true porto-systemic shunt was performed. A certain French surgeon, Léon Émile Vidal (1834–1926), from the town of Périgueux in the Dordogne, actually performed the first end-to-side portocaval shunt for hematemesis, which he reported in 1903. Vidal apparently knew about and followed precisely the experimental method of portocaval shunt outlined by the Italian Iginio Tansini from Palermo. By 1902, Tansini had perfected his technique of anastomosis of splanchnic end of the portal vein to the side of the inferior vena cava using fine silk sutures on cadavers and then successfully carried out the anastomosis in several dogs [18].[3] Vidal's patient survived the operation but succumbed 4 months later from some type of endovascular infection, for which Vidal then condemned the principle of the operation (his portocaval shunt) [19].[4]

Yet further improvements were to come. The accomplished French surgeon Alexis Carrel described a refined technique for performing the *fistule d'Eck* in 1906, first aligning the inferior vena cava just above entrance of the renal veins with the portal vein. Both were then occluded by *bandelettes de toile* (cloth strips), and 15 mm cuts were made in each vessel. The anastomosis was then completed with a simple running suture. Following completion the portal vein was then ligated immediately as it left the liver. His technique was well tolerated by the experimental animals [20].[5] Little more was done in the way of porto-systemic shunting until the

---

[3] Iginio Tansini (1855–1943) would achieve more notoriety for his work in developing the musculocutaneous latissimus dorsi flap to cover defects created by the radical mastectomy.

[4] Vidal seemed still very much enamored with the omentopexy of Drummond and Morison, but apparently was unable to do it in this particular case, at which time he tried his innovative portal vein to side of vena cava anastomosis.

[5] Carrel was later awarded the Nobel Prize in Physiology or Medicine for his innovative techniques in vascular suturing.

landmark paper of Alan Whipple at Columbia- Presbyterian Hospital in New York City in 1945 in which he described his experience with ten patients suffering from "Banti's disease" (portal hypertension and splenomegaly/hypersplenism) on whom he performed either a splenic vein to left renal vein (five) or an end-to-side portal vein to inferior vena cava (five).[6] In each he used the vitallium tubes as a sutureless conduit as perfected by Arthur Blakemore and Jere Lord, two faculty members at the same institution. All ten patients survived the operation with significant clinical improvement in at least five [22]. In 1946, before the first meeting of Edward Churchill's Excelsior Surgical Club, Alfred Blalock gave a lecture on performance of vascular shunts in cases of portal hypertension. As opposed to Whipple's group, Blalock preferred the suturing technique, believing patency rates were superior (although his experience was not near that of Whipple and colleagues) [23].[7]

In fact others had become enamored with surgery for portal hypertension. Skilled surgeon Charles G. Child III, while at New York-Cornell, wrote extensively on the subject, describing in great detail perturbations of anatomy and physiology brought about by obstruction to portal flow, either within or outside the liver. He was an advocate of either splenorenal shunts (extra-hepatic portal obstruction) or end-to-side portocaval shunts in selected patients with portal hypertension. In his major tome on portal hypertension Child summarized the world experience of portocaval shunting up to that time, compiling 362 cases, the majority done between 1950 and 1954. Immediate postoperative mortality was 14 percent but late results were largely unknown. Child was free to say, however, based on his personal experience.

> It is apparent, then, from these data that patients in whom an effective decrease in portal pressure was obtained have not bled again. … Furthermore, it is obvious … that the porta-caval anastomosis, while effectively lowering the pressure in the portal bed, does not materially affect the progressive course of cirrhosis [25].[8]

It was soon learned that overall survival in these patients did not substantially improve. Instead, progressive liver failure was the usual course, as if the liver, now deprived of nutrient portal blood, accelerated its downward spiral with worsening hepatocyte function until basic metabolic processes were unsustainable. It was an imperfect systemic solution to a problem totally hepatic. By 1960, others, like Arthur Blakemore, fully agreed with Child and freely admitted that life expectancy was determined by the cirrhosis, not portal hypertension [27].

---

[6] The term "portal hypertension" seemed to originate from a report in 1906 by Parisians Augustin Gilbert and Maurice Villaret describing the origins of ascites in cirrhotic livers: "for us ascites is a function of the syndrome of portal hypertension [*d'hypertension portale*]" [21].

[7] For a fascinating discussion of the early work of Whipple, Blakemore, and Blalock I direct you to the superb article by W. Dean Warren [24].

[8] Charles Child (1908–1991) together with colleague Jerome Turcotte and, later, the Britain Nicholas Pugh devised a scoring system to determine liver reserve in anticipation of porto-systemic shunting in portal hypertension. This scoring system has been applied in general as a prognostic aid in chronic (cirrhotic) liver disease only of late to be supplanted by the Model for End Stage Liver Disease (MELD) scoring to more accurately prioritize recipients for liver transplantation. See Ref. [26].

12.2   The Formidable Operation: Unspoken Alliances

It was this observation, perhaps, that prompted a young Thomas Starzl to envision the ultimate solution: total liver replacement. His experiences while in training at the University of Miami under Dean Warren were etched deep:

> There is no more terrifying sight in medicine than an ashen and panic-stricken patient, bleeding internally into the esophagus and stomach and then vomiting his life's blood onto the floor before anything can be done to help (see [1], p 55).

At once curiosity overtook him. In his spare time he set up an animal lab in an empty garage across from Jackson Memorial Hospital. The technical aspects were daunting. As a first step he perfected a method for hepatectomy and studied the effects of an anhepatic state on dogs.[9] Starzl then turned his attention to the second step: sewing in a new liver. It was tedious, repetitious, and discouraging effort. Having moved to Chicago with a fellowship in thoracic surgery he continued his liver work in his spare time. There was no deterring him, even with his faculty appointment at Northwestern University. Even after technical aspects of liver removal and implantation had been mastered, he faced a new challenge: preservation of the explanted homograft. How would he preserve liver tissue totally deprived of blood flow and oxygen until it could be transplanted in another host? The challenge was monumental. In Chicago he began experimenting with the new concept of hypothermia that had been introduced by colleagues John Lewis and Norman Shumway.[10] One has to only understand the relentless energy, unfathomable tenacity, and uncompromising conviction of Thomas Starzl to envision any hope of success.

But he was not alone. Francis Moore (1913–2001), Chief of Surgery at Harvard's Peter Bent Brigham Hospital in Boston, developed an early interest in transplantation, working along with colleague David Hume.[11] By 1957 Moore had recruited a young crew of residents that included Brownell "Brownie" Wheeler to work out schemes for liver transplantation in dogs. From Moore's perspective, the liver represented a huge antigen load such that, he thought, if transplanted it could stun the immune system into inactivity. More or less, passive allograft acceptance. His team began their laboratory work a few weeks later. As Starzl well knew, there were immediate technical challenges that awaited such a prodigious operation. Despite early discouraging results, Moore's group was eventually able to get a few survivors

---

[9] The "anhepatic phase" represents that period of time when the liver has been removed and the new homograft (allograft) has not yet been implanted. During that time the host suffers from deprivation of all liver function (primarily clotting and detoxifying abilities) and adequate blood flow, as all portal and systemic (inferior vena cava) blood has been clamped off.

[10] F. John Lewis (1916–1993) and Norman Shumway (1923–2006) were introduced at the University of Minnesota in the early 1950s. Shumway, in particular, began his study of the effects of hypothermia on organ preservation for heart transplantation some years later at Stanford University [28].

[11] David Hume (1917–1973) was a transplant pioneer in his own right. After training at Harvard Hume was appointed the Stuart McGuire Professor and Chairman of Surgery at the Medical College of Virginia in 1956 where he continued his work in renal transplantation. His untimely death in 1973 was the result of an airplane crash in California.

after "one-stage homotransplantations." The most precise and delicate techniques were required, including the use of venous shunts to divert systemic and portal blood pent up during the anhepatic phase. "Survival has been gratifying although very exacting demands are made on surgical technique for its achievement," Moore went on to say, capsulizing a most frustrating experience getting dogs through the operation [29].[12] In 1960, Moore's group reported their results to the American Surgical Association annual meeting. Of the 31 animals transplanted, 15 survived over 24 h and 8 lived for several days [30].

While Starzl and Moore achieved wide notoriety for their efforts in liver transplantation, they were not the first to attempt this. In the early 1950s, Stuart Welch at Albany Medical College had already reported some success in dogs with heterotopic, auxiliary (piggy-back) liver transplantation. Survival was enhanced, in Welch's opinion, by providing both arterial and venous inflow to the donor liver, by way of a non-splanchnic venous source. There were 47 attempts with 14 "successes." Survivability extended until, presumably, immunologic rejection of the organ occurred several days later, essentially reducing the grafted liver to a "small shrunken remnant of barely recognizable liver tissue." Despite his technical achievements, Welch was sanguine about the future of such surgery, even without the specter of immunologic attack [31][13]:

> It is interesting to speculate about the possibility of transplanting the human liver in part or as a whole. The two problems of donation and the technique of operation seem by themselves to be insurmountable obstacles with our present knowledge.

In fact, Welch had missed a critical understanding. His two livers had different sources for portal flow, the native liver, of course, by way of the portal circulation, and the auxiliary liver by way of the systemic circulation. The small, shrunken liver remnant described by Welch may not have been an immunologic phenomenon as much as deprivation of portal blood, and therefore—at least in Starzl's mind as he related later—hepatotrophic factors (see [1], p 126).

Starzl would carry his passion to the extreme. In an almost manic endeavor to surmount the intricacies of liver replacement, he would perform transplants on over 200 canines. By 1960, Starzl's dogs were faring just as well as Moore's, many surviving the formidable operation of liver removal and replacement and living at least a few days. At the American Surgical Association meeting in West Virginia in 1960 he and Moore met. "It was clear," Moore later wrote, "we were working in parallel … We enjoyed a congenial relationship, not one of rivalry," critical, Moore believed, for the advance of science in this new field of transplantation [32].

But it was Starzl who first tried this stupendous operation in humans. Despite discouraging public comments like those of Nobel Laureate Sir Frank Burnet in 1961 that "the present outlook [for genetically dissimilar donor-recipient] is highly

---

[12] All quotes taken from this publication.

[13] C. Stuart Welch (1909–1980) was Professor of Surgery at Albany Medical College. While his work on auxiliary liver transplantation met with early failure, the concept was vital to an understanding of the role of portal blood in engrafted livers. As Starzl later said "[w]hat Welch had done without knowing it was to create an experimental model of enormous power" (see [1], p 126).

unfavorable to success" [33], on March 1, 1963, Starzl embarked on the first human liver transplantation—in a child with biliary atresia. The boy exsanguinated on the table from a combination of dense abdominal adhesions and fibrinolysis from his end-stage liver disease. Despite this setback, hardly noticed in the press, Starzl's second attempt was a resounding success. The patient had been found to harbor multiple nodules of hepatocellular carcinoma in his cirrhotic liver. In contrast to the one-stage operation attempted on the child, the second patient had a two-stage oper-ation: first only skeletonizing all vascular structures in and out of the liver in an attempt to minimize the disastrous blood loss of his first case. The patient was closed and returned to the ward. Just short of 1 day later he was taken back to the operating room for liver removal and homotransplantations. One observer reported the following day that "It seemed to me that the patient was in better shape than the surgeons on the day after this monumental effort" (see [1], p 103). The patient lived a total of 7 days. By the end of 1963, Starzl had reported three cases of human orthotopic liver transplantation; his third patient suffering from an intrahepatic chol-angiocarcinoma also survived the operation and lasted 22 days [34].

Just as in his dogs technical problems with donor and recipient would plague Starzl's early efforts, magnified many times in humans. Removal of the recipient native liver was often thwarted by massive varices from cirrhosis-induced portal hypertension, producing catastrophic blood loss. The anhepatic phase itself required liberal blood transfusions to the upper torso to maintain sufficient cardiac output, venous return from the lower body barricaded by clamps on the portal and inferior vena cava systems. And then there was the uncertainty of allograft viability and adequate tissue preservation to begin functioning at once following reperfusion. The whole process was fraught with tension and anxiety in those early days. And in the back of everyone's mind was the nagging question: should we be doing this at all?

Ethical concerns were aggravated by Jean Demirleau's experience in France. In 1964, Demirleau performed the first liver transplant in Europe in Paris at the *Hôpital* Saint-Antoine, the same institution that had fostered the pioneering efforts of André Bergeret, Jacques Hepp, and Jacques Caroli. His recipient was a 75-year-old patient with metastatic liver cancer (colon) and the donor a 71-year-old patient who had suffered cardiac arrest. Roughly following Starzl's technique, the operation was completed within 4 h but the patient died 3 h later, apparently from irreversible bleeding due to fibrinolysis—almost certainly an ischemic liver implant little inclined to function. Once again, this elaborate procedure had failed, donor and recipient much too old and sick to withstand surgery of this magnitude [35].[14]

Nevertheless, now Starzl had become obsessed with transplantation, convinced that technical problems could be overcome and widely publishing his results and

---

[14] In his report, Demirleau freely admitted he did not follow the technique of Starzl in performing the recipient hepatectomy nor in decompressing the portal system during the anhepatic and engrafting phase. Actually and critically, preservation of the donor liver in Demirleau's case seemed inadequate and consisted of only topical cooling in the donor whereas Starzl provided cooled oxygenated perfused blood throughout the donor phase instituted immediately after pro-nouncement of death [36].

observations. Work was unrelenting, and cigarettes were his indulgence. Twenty-four hours stints of operating, rounding, and writing demanded it, he felt. Starzl scrutinized his bailiwick with stealthy insomnia and ruminated on the mysteries of immunology at each patient's door. With lips pursed, eyes riveted, cigarette at the ready Starzl scoured his patient's "wall-charts," looking for clues of success or failure, knowing that somewhere in those numbers lay the secrets of allograft tolerance. And it was such ponderings that consumed him and forced from him an unrelenting energy to part the curtain of certitude and lay bare those vast regions of the unexplored. It was here that the genius felt most at home. It was here that he knew he must reside. In the operating room, with the same intensity, he parsed delicate structures in the porta hepatis or sutured minute vessels with fine silk. There was no "flash" in his demeanor, just steady, focused labor, as if an intense and unseen struggle had ensued between his mortal talents and the occult and defiant forces of nature. By 1967, there had been nine attempts at human orthotopic liver transplantation, seven done in Denver by Starzl's group, and one each in Boston (the patient lived but 11 days) and Paris (Demirleau's effort at Saint-Antoine)—both of these immediately unsuccessful. Then in a 4-month period in 1967 Starzl's group performed four more, all of whom survived the operation, three living more than 1 month [37]. By 1970, his team had carried out 216 kidney and more than 30 liver transplants. By the end of his tenure in Denver, Starzl had performed over 150 liver transplants. Yet chronic rejection, technical problems, and, very likely, inadequate tissue preservation contributed to high attrition. One year patient survival was still below 50% [38].

The wonder drug cyclosporine would change all that. Survival would soar and others, worldwide, would follow Starzl's lead. And it all began with the curiosity of a bright young British surgeon.

Roy Calne, that bright young surgeon, had become intrigued with transplantation of organs after hearing a lecture by fellow Brit Peter Medawar on immunologic tolerance. Calne had come from simple means, his father a mechanical engineer with rural roots. Roy himself was described as a "rebellious youth" who chose medicine over engineering but lacked the marks for an education at Cambridge or Oxford and, instead, took a position at Guy's Hospital Medical School. There, he became enamored with surgery and the practical black-or-white issues it presented. "Surgical evidence," he would say, "[t]here was no way of arguing against it."[15] Yet, he was also intrigued by the theoretical, the unproven. Calne was captivated by the immune system and its ability to reject anything foreign. Could it be modified to allow transplantation from one individual to another? But even the brilliant Medawar was pessimistic. During that same lecture, when asked about what applications of his experimental work there could be to actual patient treatment, Medawar paused for a moment and then firmly replied "Absolutely none."

Well, Calne was not so convinced. He took the novel drug 6-mercaptopurine to the laboratory and used it on dogs after kidney transplantation. It worked. Rejection

---

[15] Interview with Sir Roy Calne by Dr. Max Blythe, Trinity Hall, Cambridge, December 13, 1996: The Royal College of Physicians and Oxford Brooks University Medical Sciences Video Archive MSVA 154.

was abrogated, work that caught the attention of Medawar and led to a yearlong sabbatical in the United States [39]. Calne secured a spot with Francis Moore in his Boston laboratory in 1960. It would be strictly "bench" research. There was little enthusiasm for clinical application in those days. When Calne had inquired about transplanting a kidney to a hopelessly ill patient, he was bluntly told "It can't be done." Little deterred by this pessimism Calne set out to understand the major barrier—that profound and deep-seated immune attack on any implanted foreign tissue.[16]

But even before that quest, there were methodological problems to surmount. The very act of connecting artery and veins in kidneys and livers demanded the utmost diligence and attention to detail. It was in Boston that Calne was first exposed to the tedious work of liver replacement. Back in London he began further work in kidney grafting. After taking charge of the surgical services at Cambridge and setting up practice at Addenbrooke's Hospital,[17] he switched his attention to the liver, working with the pig model to perfect his technique of implantation—based on the procedures set forth by Moore and Starzl—and finally obtained consistent short-term survivals [41]. In 1967, Calne performed the first British liver transplant in a desperately ill patient with alcoholic cirrhosis. It did not go well. The donor liver suffered from prolonged warm ischemia and failed to function promptly. The patient hemorrhaged after implantation and never regained consciousness. He died within 24 h [42].

A second transplant over 1 year later was on an infant with biliary atresia. While the transplant was technically successful, the child suddenly arrested after surgery and could not be resuscitated. A patient with cholangiocarcinoma was the third case and lived 11 months after transplantation even with a partially infarcted liver homograft. Case four was successful with survival exceeding several weeks. Case five died after 3 weeks. The extreme urgency and moribund condition of the recipients combined with marginal cold preservation of the donor liver provided outcomes that were disheartening, yet Calne remained optimistic. The technical factors could be worked out, he reasoned. And anyway only so much experience could be garnished from laboratory animals. Yet opposition from his colleagues mounted. In discussing further human liver transplants "they all gave their verdict, and it was universally negative" he later told a reporter. "They each had different reasons, but nobody wanted to do it."[18] Only the serendipitous presence of Dr. Francis Moore, at

---

[16] Quotes from Hurst [40]; while in Boston Calne trialed a new drug, later called azathioprine (Imuran) to provide immunosuppression. It was this drug Moore and colleague Joseph Murray used in their first unrelated human kidney transplant in 1962 (Moore, *A Miracle and a Privilege*, 180–182).

[17] Calne was appointed Chair of Surgery at Cambridge in 1965, a position that he claimed, in his self-effacing fashion, was not terribly sought after because it paid less than other university chairs (Interview with Sir Roy Calne by Dr. Max Blythe, Trinity Hall, Cambridge, December 13, 1996: Royal College of Physicians and Oxford Brooks University Medical Sciences Video Archive MSVA 154).

[18] Calne interview, December 13, 1996, Royal College of Surgeons Video Archive.

Cambridge for a collegial visit, swayed the crowd, "this is the most perfect opportunity to proceed and we've got to do it," Moore piped in. The audience suddenly quieted. Moore's reputation had preceded him. "He broke the opposition completely," Calne remembered. Consent was granted. The next transplant was successful, and the child lived 2 months, but this was a springboard for more trials, and further successes came—albeit grudgingly.

Calne's efforts bolstered Starzl's struggling program in Denver, and by 1969 33 liver transplants had been performed worldwide.[19] "The fate of liver transplantation would depend on an unspoken trans-Atlantic alliance between Cambridge and Denver without which further efforts could not have continued," Starzl later commented [43]. Calne's experience with the new drug cyclosporine was absolutely unbelievable. Use in kidney transplantation had produced startling results. Starzl wanted it, and by their close collaboration, the first United States center to trial it was Starzl's at the University of Pittsburgh Medical Center.[20] The two, Starzl and Calne, would be likened to a modern-day Cosmas and Damian, the medieval surgeon-saints who, it was said, transplanted a gangrenous leg from a recently deceased soldier. Their pursuit would be every bit as daunting as those mythical surgeons of the past millennia—to preserve and connect an organ from another human and to quiet the stubborn immune response. But surmount they did, perfecting the mechanistic and the humoral. Within mere decades "Calne and Starzl persevered, converting liver transplantation from a divinely inspired miracle into a marvel of science" [40].

Of course little progress could occur in removing deceased donor organs, transporting some distance, and then reimplanting them unless there was an ability to preserve cellular function in the meantime. Once blood flow ceased, the dying process began, and in short order, irreversible changes would occur that precluded organ function when blood flow was established in the recipient—what would later be called "reperfusion injury." Tissue preservation was key. And the science of organ preservation is almost synonymous with Folkert Belzer (1930–1995). The cerebral Dr. Belzer had begun work on organ preservation while at the University of California—San Francisco in the 1960s during the early days of deceased donor kidney transplantation. Similar efforts in those days to preserve the liver by the same methods met with disappointing failure. The routine method of preservation was immediate flushing with a chilled electrolyte solution, storage on ice, and fast transport and transplantation (the so-called "cold storage" method). For livers this meant precise coordination of donor and recipient operations and, in the early days in Denver, chartered jet travel. In fact, it was not unusual to fly the entire donor to Denver, recover the liver, and fly the body back. In those early days in Denver,

---

[19] In fact, a worldwide moratorium on liver transplantation was voluntarily enforced in 1963. During that time work continued in Starzl's Denver laboratories on evaluation of the auxiliary transplant technique, organ preservation, and new immunosuppressive drugs (prednisone, azathioprine, and anti-lymphocyte sera—key items, all felt, in successfully transplanting and maintaining allografts. Starzl resumed his human liver transplants in 1967.

[20] For a discussion of how this all was arranged, see [1], p 210–213.

Starzl's trusted recovery surgeon Charlie Halgrimson (1934–2013), invariably ready for travel at a moment's notice, became a proficient retrieval surgeon but insisted on first-class accommodations for his efforts (to the distinct enjoyment of his accompanying fellows).

Yet, even with this technique, cold storage of livers often damaged sinusoidal endothelium and resulted in variable perfusion of the organ with reimplantation. Keen to investigate, Belzer fiddled in his lab, his pipe invariably dangling from his mouth as if the two were habitually fused. With his move to the University of Wisconsin as Chairman of Surgery in 1974 work continued, adding and subtracting chemicals in the tiny laboratory afforded him. By pouring over the Merck Index and Sigma-Aldrich catalog,[21] he and his coworker James Southard finally decided on two acidic forms of saccharides, gluconic acid and lactobionic acid as ionic macromolecules that would impede the cellular swelling which seemed to occur with cold storage—that and approximating the bathing solution to intracellular electrolyte content. So, Belzer and Southard added electrolytes and other agents until, in Belzer's estimation, they had created the "kitchen sink" perfusate (he tongue-in-cheek remarked that it contained everything but the kitchen sink). Introduced in 1984 as the University of Wisconsin (UW) solution, it revolutionized organ preservation, including livers, somehow stabilizing cellular membranes and retarding cellular swelling. Immediate allograft function was impressive even with 24 h of cold storage. Much of the angst of ischemic damage from cold storage of livers had been eliminated.[22] There is no doubt that the steady improvement in success with liver transplantation was multifactorial—better patient selection, better immunosuppression—but there is little doubt that a major contributing factor was Belzer's "kitchen sink" perfusate.

There would be other European attempts. Rudolf Pichlmayr (1932–1997) was a gifted young surgeon born in Munich. He had trained in his hometown under the fabled Rudolf Zenker (1903–1984). There he was inspired by a lecture from William Kolff and developed an interest in organ replacement, working then with Professor Walter Brendel in transplant immunology. Together with American-trained thoracic surgeon Hans Borst, Pichlmayr developed an anti-lymphocytes serum that showed promise in blunting acute rejection. In 1968, Borst and Pichlmayr moved to the *Medizinischen Hochschule* in Hannover (Medical University of Hannover) to develop a new department of surgery, with emphasis on organ transplantation. That same year Pichlmayr's group performed the first kidney transplant. Between 1972 and 1977 that same transplant team at the *Medizinischen Hochschule* headed by Pichlmayr performed seven liver transplants. The first patient 19 years old survived only days, dying of "cardiopulmonary failure" but the second case was successful,

[21] The Merck Index is a literal encyclopedia of chemicals, drugs, and biologic agents published by the Royal Society of Chemistry. The Sigma-Aldrich catalog, produced by MilliporeSigma of Saint Louis, is a similar compendium of organic and inorganic chemicals.

[22] See Folkert O. Belzer, "Organ Preservation: A Personal Perspective" at https://web.stanford.edu/dept/HPST/transplant/html/belzer.html. Accessed February 3, 2020.

the patient, with a primary liver cancer, lived beyond 2 years. Of the next five, three lived beyond 2 months [44].[23]

On January 6, 1978, Henri Bismuth and his team at the *Hôpital* Paul Brousse transplanted a liver from a 5-year-old child into a 49-year-old man with fulminant Hepatitis B. The liver was placed as an auxiliary transplant because of the size discrepancy, and flow was reestablished via the vena cava, portal vein, and hepatic artery. With triple therapy immunosuppression the patient recovered and was alive 28 months after transplant [47]. Bismuth had previously transplanted four patients desperately ill with end-stage liver disease. His results had been dismal. Three of the four had promptly died. The fourth survived but was re-transplanted 10 months after the first with a split-liver allograft (right lobe) used as an auxiliary liver transplant. His conclusion was succinct. Near terminal patients with deteriorating organ function could not survive transplantation. Less ill, but still irreversibly damaged by cirrhosis, represented a more favorable group who could survive this formidable operation [48].[24] His experience over a 10 year period up to the end of 1984 was not much better. One-fifth of his patients survived a year and little more than 10 percent 2 years. However, from 1984 to 1987, with the introduction of cyclosporine results dramatically improved. Of the next 125 transplants 107 were still alive, a survival rate of 85% [49].

And by 1989 Starzl had become convinced of the utility of liver transplantation in clinical medicine. Leaving Denver in 1980 had put Starzl's entire liver program on hold but now in Pittsburgh and armed with the wonder drug Cyclosporine, his program flourished, now in Pittsburgh his program flourished, producing hundreds of liver transplants per year. Buoyed by his confidence and success, liver transplant centers blossomed at a number of European centers—Rudolf Pichlmayr in Hannover, Henri Bismuth in Paris, and Ruud Krom in Groningen—establishing the all-important "generalizability" of this treatment for end-stage liver disease and primary liver cancer.[25] The only impediments seemed to be financing and donor supply [50]. Yet, philosophically, there was no doubt that "[t]he conceptual appeal of liver transplantation is so great that the procedure may come to mind as a last resort for virtually every patient with lethal hepatic disease," the annual need for liver transplantation, he calculated at that time, was 15 per million population (figures from [51]). However, suitable deceased donors were precious few.

A possible solution was suggested by Rudolf Pichlmayr in 1989 with his report of a split-liver transplant. The donor liver was split in two, the topographical left lobe (segments II and III) transplanted into a child and the topographical right lobe

---

[23] Further information on Rudolph Pichlmayr from Christoph Broelsch [45], and Konrad Messmer [46]. Hans Borst would become a pioneer in thoracic surgery, performing the first heart transplant in Hannover in 1983 and the first combined heart-lung transplant in Germany in 1987.

[24] Without a doubt cyclosporine had revolutionized liver transplantation, and indeed transplantation in general.

[25] Ruud Krom, a disciple of Starzl's, having studied under him in Denver, performed the first liver transplant in Groningen, The Netherlands, in 1979. Until 1983 when he moved to the Mayo Clinic, he and his team did 26 more with survival rates exceeding 60% at 2 years.

into an adult [52].[26] Could this be utilized more often to ease the donor shortage? Early experience on a larger scale was questionable. In 1990, the transplant team at the University of Chicago reported higher mortality in adults with split-liver allografts and lower overall graft survival. It was their opinion that split-liver grafting should not be done in adults [55]. And, indeed, subsequent experience has borne this out. From a single-center report (UCLA) in 2009 60% of split-liver grafts were used in children. In total this comprised one-quarter of pediatric liver donors as compared to 3% of adult recipients receiving a split-liver graft [56]. As of 2015 data generated by the United States Organ Procurement and Transplantation Network indicated that of the 113,394 deceased donor liver transplants since 1995 1546 (1.36%) were split-liver grafts, 93% of which were transplanted into children. The Network, in this 2016 white paper, "supports all reasonable efforts to increase the number of transplants safely performed. Changes in allocation and practice to encourage split-liver transplantation are a potential means to that end."[27]

References

1. Starzl TE (1992) The puzzle people. University of Pittsburgh Press, Pittsburgh, p 54
2. Balducci GS et al (2016) A short history of portal hypertension and of its management. J Gastroenterol Hepatol 31:541–545
3. Brown J (1685) A remarkable account of a liver, appearing glandulous to the eye. Phil Trans R Soc 178:1266–1268
4. Baillie M (1793) Morbid anatomy of some of the Most important parts of the human body. J. Johnson, London, pp 141–142
5. Laennec RT (1819) De l'auscultation médiate. Brosson et Chaude, Paris, pp 368–369
6. Osler W (1892) *The principles and practice of medicine*. D. Appleton and Company, New York, p 441
7. Duffin JM (1987) Why does cirrhosis belong to Laennec? CMAJ 137:393–396
8. Oré M (1856) Influence de l'Oblitération de la Veine Porte sur la Sécrétion de la Bile et sur la Fonction Glycogénique du Foie. Compt rend séances Acad Sci 43:463–467
9. Logan JP, Westmoreland WF (1857) Obliteration of the portal vein and the secretion of bile. Atlanta Med Surg J 2:379–381
10. Kiernan F (1833) The anatomy and physiology of the liver. Phil Trans R Soc A 123:711–770
11. Lautenbach BF (1877) On a new function of the liver. Philadelphia Med Times 7:387–394
12. Child CG (1953) Eck's fistula. Surg Gynecol Obstet 96:374–376
13. Hahn MM et al (1893) Die Eck'sche Fistel zwischen der unteren Hohlvene und der Pfortader und ihre Folgen für den Organismus. Arch Exp Pathol Pharmakol 32:161–210
14. Whipple GH, Sperry JA (1909) Chloroform poisoning, liver necrosis and repair. Johns Hopkins Hosp Bull 20:278–289

---

[26] Actually Bismuth's group first reported using a "reduced-size" liver graft in a child (adult left lobe) in 1984 [53]. They then reported the use of split livers (separated down Cantlie's line) in 1989 in two adult patients with fulminant hepatitis. While each survived the operation they both died within 2 months of infectious complications [54].

[27] "Split Versus Whole Liver Transplantation", Organ Procurement and Transplantation Network, December, 2016, DHS https://optn.transplant.hrsa.gov/resources/ethics/split-versus-whole-liver-transplantation/ accessed July 3, 2019.

15. Sappey MC (1883) Mémoire sur les Veines Portes Accessoire. J l'Anat et Physiol 19:517–524
16. Talma S (1898) Chirurgische oeffnung neuer seitenbahnen für das blut der vena porta. Klin Woschenschr 35:833–836
17. Drummond DM (1896) A case of ascites due to cirrhosis of the liver cured by operation. Br Med J 2:728–729
18. Tansini I (1902) Ableitung des Portalen Blutes Durch die Direkte Verbindung der V. Portae mit der V. Cava, Neus Operatives. Zentralblatt fur Chirurgie 29:937–939
19. Vidal M (1903) Traitement chirurgicale des ascites. Presse Med 11:747
20. Carrel A, Guthrie C-C (1906) Méthode Simple Pour Établir Une Fistule d'Eck. Compt rendus seances Soc Biol fil 60:1104–1106
21. Gilbert AV, Villaret M (1906) Contribution a l'Etude du Syndrome d'Hypertension Portale. Comptes rendus Soc biol 60:820–821
22. Whipple AO (1945) The problem of portal hypertension in relation to the hepatosplenopathies. Ann Surg 122:449–475
23. Blalock A (1947) The use of shunt or by-pass operations in the treatment of certain circulatory disorders, including portal hypertension and pulmonic stenosis. Ann Surg 125:129–141
24. Warren WD (1980) Reflections on the early development of portacaval shunts. Ann Surg 191:519–527
25. Child CG III (1954) The hepatic circulation and portal hypertension. W.B. Saunders Co., Philadelphia, pp 222–265, quote 242
26. Child CG, Turcotte JG (1964) Surgery and portal hypertension. In: Child CG (ed) The liver and portal hypertension. W.B. Saunders Co., Philadelphia, pp 50–64
27. Blakemore AH (1958) Nutritional requirements and management in patients with cirrhosis of the liver pre- and postoperatively. Ann Surg 147:875–881
28. Baumgartner WA et al (2009) Norman E. SHumway, MD, PhD: visionary, innovator, humorist. J Thoracic Cardiovasc Surg 137:269–277
29. Moore FD et al (1959) One-stage homotransplantation of the liver following total hepatectomy in dogs. Transplant Bull 6:103–107
30. Moore FD et al (1960) Experimental whole-organ transplantation of the liver and of the spleen. Ann Surg 152:374–385
31. Welch S (1955) A note on transplantation of the whole liver in dogs. Transplant Bull 2:54–55
32. Moore FD (1995) A miracle and a privilege. Joseph Henry Press, Washington DC, p 190
33. Burnet FM (1961) The new approach to immunology. N Engl J Med 264:24–34
34. Starzl TE et al (1963) Homotransplantation of the liver in humans. Surg Gynecol Obstet 117:659–676
35. Demirleau JN et al (1964) Tentative d'Homogreffe Hépatique. Mem Acad Chir (Paris) 90:177–179
36. Maggi U, Azoulay D (2013) Further details from the first human liver transplantation in Europe. Transplantation 96:e47–e48
37. Starzl TE et al (1968) Extended survival in 3 cases of orthotopic homotransplantation of the liver. Surgery 63:549–563
38. Starzl TE et al (1979) Fifteen years of clinical liver transplantation. Gastroenterology 77:375–388
39. Calne RY (1960) The rejection of renal homografts. Inhibition in dogs by 6-Mercaptopurine. Lancet 1:417–418
40. Hurst J (2012) A modern day Cosmas and Damian: sir Roy Calne and Thomas Starzl receive the 2012 Lasker-Debakey clincial medical research award. J Clin Invest 122:3378–3382
41. Calne RY et al (1967) Observations of orthotopic liver transplantation in the pig. BMJ 2:478–480
42. Calne RY (1968) Liver transplantation in man—I, observations on technique and organization in five cases. BMJ 4:535–540
43. Busuttil RW, Klintmalm BG (2014) Transplantation of the liver. Elsevier Health Sciences, Philadelphia

44. Schaps DH (1978) Zur Orthotopen Lebertransplantation aus Anaesthesiologischer Sicht. Anaesthesist 27:405–415
45. Broelsch C (1990) In memory of Rudolph Pichlmayr, MD, FRCS, FACS. Liver Transplant Surg 4:116–118
46. Messmer K (1998) Prof. Dr. Rudolph Pichlmayr, 1932-1997. European Surg Res 30:77–78
47. Houssin DB et al (1980) Heterotopic liver transplantation in end-stage HBsAg-positive cirrhosis. Lancet 1:990–993
48. Houssin DF et al (1980) Criteria for hepatic transplantation in cirrhosis. Surg Gynecol Obstet 151:30–32
49. Bismuth H (1988) Liver transplantation: the Paul Brousse experience. Transplant Proc 20:486–488
50. Rigter H, Bos MA (1990) The diffusion of organ transplantation in Western Europe. Health Policy 16:133–145
51. Starzl TE et al (1989) Liver transplantation (first of two parts). N Engl J Med 321:1014–1022
52. Pichlmayr RR et al (1989) Transplantation einer Spenderleber auf zwei Empfanger. Eine neue Methode in der Wetzentwicklung der Lebersegment Transplantation. Langenbecks Arch Chir 373:127–130
53. Bismuth HH et al (1984) Reduced-sized Orthotopic liver graft in hepatic transplantation in children. Surgery 95:367–370
54. Bismuth HM et al (1989) Emergency orthotopic liver transplantation in two patients using one donor liver. Br J Surg 76:722–724
55. Broelsch CE et al (1990) Application of reduced-size liver transplants as split grafts, auxiliary orthotopic grafts, and living related segmental transplants. Ann Surg 212:368–377
56. Hong JC (2009) Longterm outcomes for whole and segmental liver grafts in adult and pediatric liver transplant recipients: a 10-year comparative analysis of 2,988 cases. J Am Coll Surg 208:682–691

Chapter 13
Splitting the Soul

In parallel with efforts to replace the entire organ, surgeons would become embold-ened to split this divine structure—almost deified as lodging for the soul itself by contemplative ancients—in any number of innovative manners. Starzl's passion for transplantation only engendered a mounting curiosity and mastery of the partial hepatectomy. During those early years of liver allografting, he and his team per-formed 27 liver resections including 14 "trisegmentectomies," or what had formerly been called topographic right lobectomies—without a single postoperative death. Starzl referred to this operation as removal of the "true right lobe" plus the medial segment of the "true" left lobe—terms synonymous with right and left livers of Couinaud, split by the interlobar plane of Cantlie. For the trisegmentectomy he used an abdominal approach, discouraging the thoracic extension that, he felt, contrib-uted significantly to postoperative morbidity.[1] Hilar control was followed by control of the right hepatic vein. "This maneuver is potentially dangerous," he wrote, "because the hepatic vein is extremely short and because a tear during the dissection would create a defect in the side of the vena cava that would be difficult to control or repair," an opinion certainly shared by anyone who has tried to force a clamp around this structure, barely visible as it emerges from liver substance to join the vena cava. Improperly done, the operating surgeon will be greeting by a seemingly unstaunchable flow of venous blood.[2] Another technical note was his insistence on leaving a margin of viable medial segment (segment IV) that is meant to preserve

---

[1] But which he would not hesitate to use—in the early days—for gigantic right-sided liver tumors.

[2] This misadventure may have dire consequences as efforts to identify the injury to the right hepatic vein will only result in more blood loss, and tamponade of this area often compromises the needed exposure to complete parenchymal transection. The liver indeed will inflict the full force of its hemorrhagic fury on the operating team.

© The Editor(s) (if applicable) and The Author(s), under exclusive license to
Springer Nature Switzerland AG 2020
T. S. Helling, D. Azoulay, *Historical Foundations of Liver Surgery*,
https://doi.org/10.1007/978-3-030-47095-1_13

nutrient vessels and biliary drainage to and from the lateral sector.[3] Splitting of the liver itself was done by crushing maneuvers with ligation of intraparenchymal branches, the same technique taught by virtually all liver surgeons before the age of hemostatic energy devices. The last structure encountered was the fat middle hepatic vein, draining the central liver, Couinaud Segments IV, V, and VIII. It was to be taken at its origin from the left hepatic vein or directly from the vena cava (all descriptions from [1]).

Starzl's technique was impeccable, total concentration and deliberate movements leaving nothing to chance or to dangerous bravado. The operating room was silent, all focused on their individual performances as part of an orchestrated recital. He demanded resolute perfection from his assistants, anesthesia, and scrub nurse. "Quickly, now," would be the icy command if there was the slightest delay in passing the right instrument or suture at a critical juncture. Only much later would Starzl reveal the pent up anxieties he faced with each operation. "I had an intense fear of failing the patients who had placed their health or life in my hands," he wrote at age 65. "I did not like to operate." So he would prepare and rehearse and review again and again and go to the operating room "sick with apprehension." His concentration there needed to be total, and thus his insistence for quiet and for order. Yet it would be this disquiet, this fear that would drive the surgeon to excel as no other before him in expanding the boundaries of liver surgery [2]. And between operative adventures he released his suppressed anxieties with wild bicycle expeditions through the Rocky Mountains up and over the Continental Divide at 11,000 feet, his faithful followers (residents and junior attendings) trailing behind.

Starzl, and Bismuth later, would become the transition liver surgeons, incorporating their confidence in transplantation, a comfort with the complexities of liver physiology, and familiarity of liver anatomy to produce an almost routine and predictable process of resection—truly Bismuth's "réglée," a term that came to mean "regulated" or "standardized." Their teams were adept at not only resection but also vascular reconstruction, born of necessity through donor hepatectomy, back bench preparation, and orthotopic insertion. And here would be the first dichotomy in liver surgery: resections would fall under the purview of transplant surgeons *and* surgical oncologists, both territorial in their belief that they alone would be eminently qualified to address tumors of the liver. Over time transplant surgeons would feel justified because of their intimate knowledge of the vascular inflow and outflow, spurred by their self-styled vascular aplomb, and the oncologists insistent that surgery be put in the holistic care often required for malignancies affecting the liver. It would pit the technical successes of transplant surgeons—complex reconstructions unimaginable a generation ago—against the evidence-based survival benefits and multi-modality treatments proposed by the oncologists.

But lest one feels that others less noticed for their transplant prowess were not adept at rearrangement of vascular anatomy; it should not be forgotten that, in 1984,

---

[3] From split-liver grafting it has been appreciated that the left hepatic duct trifurcates sending a branch to Segment IV. Compromise of this relationship could constrict biliary drainage from the left liver.

Leslie Blumgart and his team in London had completely excised the portal vein bifurcation in two patient with hilar cholangiocarcinoma, anastomosing the main portal vein to the lone remaining left branch [3]. And, in 1991, after a respite of 5 years in the medieval city of Bern, Switzerland, Professor Blumgart migrated to New York City, recruited to Memorial Sloan-Kettering Cancer Center in New York. The hospital, an amalgamation of the Memorial Cancer Hospital founded in 1884 and the endowed Sloan-Kettering Institute for Cancer Research, had engendered a culture of excellence combining strong clinical leadership with solid translational research. Here he would amass a vast experience in resectional liver surgery for neoplasms, developing many oncological practices that would be guiding principles for liver surgeons worldwide. While transplantation was not a mainstay of his practice he would acknowledge its role in the treatment of certain liver cancers. By 2001, after 10 years he and his coworkers had amassed an impressive series of 1803 liver resections, almost one-third of which were extended hepatic resections, Starzl's "trisegmentectomies." Their operative mortality was 3%, and in the last 184 resections there were no deaths. In a century of experience, liver resection, even major liver resection, had gone from a bloodied, frenzied affair to a controlled predictable operative procedure [4]. And Blumgart was the consummate champion, guiding his surgical teams to extreme measures in ridding the liver of its uninvited neoplasms. No quarter was given to the uninformed and uneducated. He was exacting in his surgical planning and merciless to those lacking the understanding, diligence, and patients to tame this dangerous organ.

So with the millennium approaching and the safety of liver resection firmly established, what would be the next frontiers in liver surgery? How much more could the human liver be manipulated, sliced, partitioned, or rearranged in order to extirpate neoplastic processes, either primary or secondary. Clearly solid cancers were still largely a surgical disease. While chemotherapeutic and targeting agents were improving and immunotherapy still in its infancy, they were not having a significant impact on bulky or multifocal hepatic lesions. Seldom was there total eradication of liver neoplasms by chemotherapy alone—and even then not necessarily a permanent condition. And all the more concerning was the systemic nature of many malignant processes. The liver often was only one manifestation of multifocal disease, not situations that favored easy—or safe—surgical solutions.[4]

From a purely technical perspective, without question transplantation had changed the face of liver surgery. The comfortable familiarity enjoyed by executing dozens of donor hepatectomies, back table preparations, and implantation of liver allografts brought about a new and daring approach to liver resection. Formerly "out of bounds" for surgeons, reordering of major liver vasculature became fertile ground for unorthodox resections. Tumors heretofore *verboten* were now fair game, tucked as they sometimes were in the crotch of hepatic veins or impinging on portal vein branches in the liver hilum. Resect and reconstruct were the guiding principles. But protection of liver parenchyma was of utmost importance. And in this

---

[4]For the impact of liver metastases in colon and rectal cancer see [5].

transplantation also contributed. An understanding of cold preservation, maintenance of cellular metabolism during times of ischemia, and protection from reperfusion injury—all underpinnings of human allograft survival—spilled over into the
realm of radical resections, interruption of major blood vessels, and the luxury of
intricate reconstruction. In 1987, little known Japanese surgeon Masatoshi Makuuchi
had reported a small group of patients with tumors involving the right hepatic vein.
Total removal of tumors along with the right hepatic vein was accomplished with a
minimum of resected liver. Venous drainage to the posterior sector was maintained
by preservation of the "minor" hepatic veins directly into the inferior vena cava. The
skill he exhibited in these procedures would shortly capture the world's attention [6]
(Fig. 13.1).

In particular, split-liver allografts refined techniques of live donor hepatectomy.
Separation of lobes had to be precise, minimizing warm ischemia and providing
sufficient length of portal vein, hepatic artery, hepatic veins, and bile ducts for anastomosis and adequate perfusion, venous drainage, and biliary channeling. Any compromise in those efforts might produce an allograft of marginal functional capacity.
Living donor hepatectomy demanded exceptional diligence, the effect on donor of
immediate concern, but also the delivery of a healthy allograft essential to success.

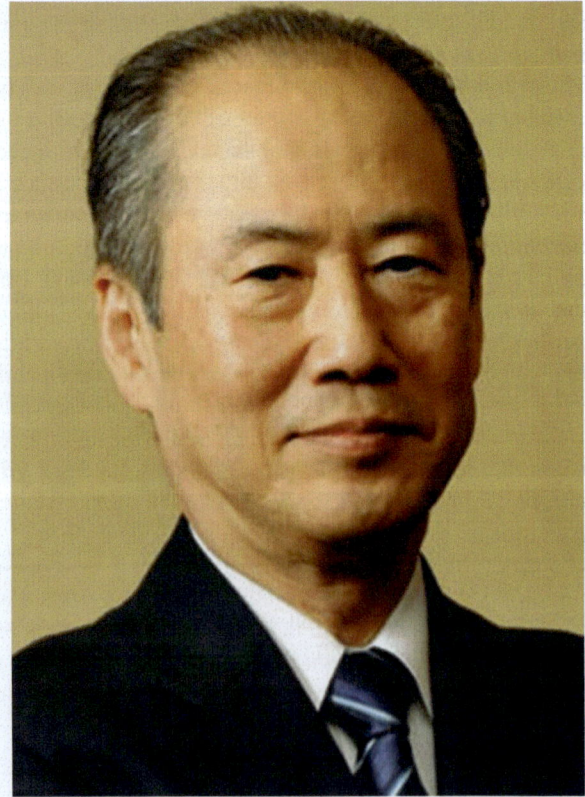

Fig. 13.1 Masatoshi
Makuuchi (American
College of Surgeons).
From Xu EX. Living
legend in surgery:
Professor Masatoshi
Makuuchi (HepatoBiliary
Surg Nutr 2015;4:303).
Photo courtesy of
M. Makuuchi

Lowering the central pressure to reduce bleeding during parenchymal dissection, use of blood scavenging equipment, understanding of patterns of venous drainage both extra-capsular and intrahepatic, and limited employment of hepatic ischemia were all desirable practices. Intraoperative ultrasound with color-flow Doppler was instrumental in mapping venous drainage to allow for preservation of veins that, if compromised, could result in segmental damage to liver parenchyma.

Such brilliance did not appear overnight. There were the occasional pioneers who, for one shining moment, unveiled methods that were purely visionary yet portended the future of hepatic strategies. Total isolation of the liver (total vascular exclusion) from all blood flow in and out had obvious advantages: a relatively bloodless field in which to dissect out tumors. In 1966, when clinical liver transplantation was still in its infancy, John Heaney and colleagues from San Antonio illustrated a technique of total vascular exclusion of the liver to facilitate completion of hepatic lobectomies. Complete control of all inflow and outflow required simultaneous clamping of portal vein and hepatic artery while the inferior vena cava was controlled inside the pericardium and above the renal veins. Such monumental efforts were tried in three patients by Heaney's group. In two patients the operations were completed successfully [7]. Joseph Fortner from the Memorial Sloan-Kettering Cancer Center in New York began experimenting with liver resection during vascular exclusion and hypothermic perfusion as early as 1970. After clamping of inferior vena cava, hepatic arterial, and portal systems, the liver was perfused through the gastroduodenal artery and branch of the portal vein to the area to be resected. The retrohepatic vena cava was vented for exit of the perfusate. In a report published in 1974 this method was tried on 29 patients with three postoperative deaths [8].[5]

By 1989, Bismuth and his team at the *Hôpital* Paul Brousse had accrued enough experience to determine that total vascular exclusion had a definite role in resection of some centrally located hepatic tumors, those in close proximity to the major hepatic veins or inferior vena cava. According to their method, clamps were applied to the inflow portal pedicle and to the inferior vena cava above (subdiaphragmatic) and below the liver. For durations of less than an hour (mean about 45 min) the liver was quite tolerant of ischemia. In this setting the operative field was essentially bloodless. Tumors could be precisely excised without damage to neighboring vascular structures. Only one of 45 patients died in the postoperative period [11]. Buoyed by this experience the group expanded their capabilities by resection and reconstruction of vascular structures—portal vein, hepatic vein, inferior vena cava, and hepatic artery—to remove tumors heretofore considered unresectable. Achievement of an oncological resection—adequate margins—and provision of enough functioning liver supplied and drained sufficiently to sustain life and initiate

---

[5] Joseph Fortner (1921–2007) practiced at Memorial Sloan-Kettering Cancer Center for over 45 years (1951–1995) and was the Chief of the Gastric and Mixed Tumor Service from 1970 to 1978. From 1970 to 1992 he personally performed 548 liver resections, and performed see Ref. [9]. In 1973 he reported his team's experience with auxiliary liver transplants in three patients, a technique that he soon abandoned [10]. Nevertheless, Dr. Fortner was a major force in hepatic and pancreatic surgery in the 1970s.

regeneration expanded their pool of potential candidates. Their results were impressive. From 1997 to 2009, 84 patients underwent these complex procedures. While the operative mortality was substantially higher than with traditional liver resections (14% versus 2%)—most due to liver failure—these were patients that had previously been considered inoperable and doomed to an early death from their metastatic disease [12].[6]

Even more unnerving was the spectacle put on by Rudolf Pichlmayr who completely removed the liver and, using hypothermic perfusion on a back table—his so-called "bench procedure"—resected bulky tumors that defied otherwise orthodox removal. Devoid of blood, the liver was more amenable to methodical, precise dissection—just as in back table splitting of livers for transplantation. If needed, rearrangement of internal vascular systems was also possible. All the while the anesthetized patient, *sans* liver, would be perfused—sometimes for hours—with veno-venous bypass. Almost unbelievably, Pichlmayr's first three cases were all successful [14]. More sobering was a follow-up report of 24 cases published in 2000. The in-hospital mortality for these convoluted undertakings (mean operative time 13 ± 3 h) was 38%, and in 10 of the survivors tumor recurrence was apparent from 13 to 36 months later. Only four patients were alive at the reporting, two of whom had resections for benign (focal nodular hyperplasia) disease [15]. The technique did not gain popularity with most surgeons. Unless there was experience in liver transplantation and familiarity with perfusion techniques the entire undertaking was simply too daunting, and the lack of effective adjuvant therapy for malignant diseases—at this point—resulted in a high likelihood of tumor reappearance.

References

1. Starzl TE et al (1975) Hepatic trisegmentectomy and other liver resections. Surg Gynecol Obstet 141:429–437
2. Starzl TE (1992) The puzzle people. University of Pittsburgh Press, Pittsburgh, p 59
3. Blumgart LH (1984) Surgical approaches to cholangiocarcinoma at confluence of hepatic ducts. Lancet 1:66–70
4. Jarnagin WR et al (2002) Improvement in perioperative outcome after hepatic resection. Ann Surg 236:397–407
5. Helling TS et al (2014) Cause of death from liver metastases in colorectal cancer. Ann Surg Oncol 21:501–506
6. Makuuchi MH et al (1987) Four new hepatectomy procedures for resection of the right hepatic vein and preservation of the inferior right hepatic vein. Surg Gynecol Obstet 164:68–72
7. Heaney JP et al (1966) An improved technic for vascular isolation of the liver: experimental study and case reports. Ann Surg 163:237–241

[6]Others were more cautious. Makuuchi's group in Tokyo avoided the use of vascular exclusion, preferring to reconstruct the cavo-hepatic junction by simple inflow occlusion. They reported no adverse events as a result. "TVE [Total Vascular Exclusion] should be restricted to exceptional patients" such as tumors infiltrating the retrohepatic inferior vena cava, they said [13].

8. Fortner JG et al (1974) Major hepatic resection using vascular isolation and hypothermic perfusion. Ann Surg 180:644–651
9. Fortner JG et al (2009) Twenty-five-year follow-up for liver resection: the personal series of Dr. Joseph G. Fortner. Ann Surg 250:908–913
10. Fortner JG et al (1973) Clinical liver heterotopic (auxiliary) transplantation. Surgery 74:739–751
11. Bismuth HC et al (1989) Major hepatic resection under total vascular exclusion. Ann Surg 210:13–19
12. Azoulay DP et al (2013) Vascular reconstruction combined with liver resection for malignant tumors. Br J Surg 100:1764–1775
13. Torzilli GM et al (2001) Liver resection without total vascular exclusion: hazardous or beneficial? Ann Surg 233:167–175
14. Pichlmayr RG (1990) Technique and preliminary results of extracorporeal liver surgery (bench procedure) and of surgery on the in situ perfused liver. Br J Surg 77:21–26
15. Oldhafer KJ et al (2000) Long-term experience after ex stiu liver surgery. Surgery 127:520–527

Chapter 14
On Regeneration

There would not be the fascination about liver surgery were it not for the fact that it is unique among human organs in its remarkable powers of restoration, a process we now call regeneration. It is not clear from a teleological standpoint why the liver possesses such properties. Some have claimed that with its central role in metabolic processes it was so endowed as to withstand the catastrophe of liver toxins in primitive mammals and primates.[1] Indeed, the structure had a spiritual quality according to ancient Greeks. Metaphysically, in antiquity, for Plato and Aristotle, the liver represented the appetitive soul, whose function was to exhibit images expressed by the rational soul, more or less "a theater of prophetic representations" [2]. Whether the story of Prometheus indicated to the ancient Greeks that the liver could regenerate is not known. There seems to be no reference to it in former writings. Neither Hippocrates nor Galen ascribed this feature to the liver [3]. It was claimed an organ of "sanguification"—the making of blood—of hemostasis, of incorporation of foodstuffs for formation of blood, but no reference to regeneration can be found. Nevertheless, the Greek word for liver, $ηπαρ$ (hepar = liver), seems to originate as a root from the word $ηπαομαι$ (hepaomai), which means "to heal" or "to mend."[2] Were there anecdotal examples of regrowth of an avulsed and exposed liver? Perhaps so, although none can be found in written literature. The earliest scientific reference may be that of French anatomist Jean Cruveihier (1791–1874) who described a condition he termed *hepar acinosum* [5]:

> It is a disease characterized by the coincidence of atrophy of the liver, which is reduced to half, one-third of its volume, and the considerable development of glandular grains. Well, in this case called cirrhosis, there is atrophy of most of the glandular grains.

---

[1] This explanation was offered by liver researcher Dr. George MIchalopoulos and Marie DeFrances in [1].

[2] Translation taken from [4].

T. S. Helling, D. Azoulay, *Historical Foundations of Liver Surgery*,
https://doi.org/10.1007/978-3-030-47095-1_14

These "*grains glanduleux*" may refer to acinar units that, in fact, were regenerating in response to atrophy of other regions of the liver.

Most early recognition of liver regrowth occurred in the setting of liver cirrhosis, where scarring and nodularity gave rise to the notion that, while certain parts of the liver shrunk (atrophied), others seemed to exhibit exuberant enlargement (hypertrophy). In other words, from autopsy observations, such cirrhotic livers could considerably exceed their normal dimensions. Microscopically, as early as 1859, formation of new connective tissue could be seen injected in and enveloping liver acini which fail to maintain their normal size and soon progressively atrophy. This mass of connective tissue was thought instrumental in creating the misshapen appearance of such diseased livers. In an extensive review of cirrhosis by Theodor Ackermann (1825–1896), pathologist at the University of Halle in Wittenberg in 1880, emphasis was placed on the explosion of connective tissue prompted by the stimulus of inflammatory disease, trapping and literally strangling individual clumps of liver cells. He used the term *leberzellenschlauch* to denote rows of liver cells, perhaps in what would later be called a sinusoidal arrangement entangled with ingrowth of persistent fibrous tissue. Regeneration, in his assessment, seemed confined to the bile ducts. Nowhere in his lengthy treatise did he address actual proliferation (*hyperplasie*) of liver cells but only connective tissue and, in some unrelated sense, biliary cells. In his estimation, the mass of liver cells gradually becomes more and more atrophic until they simply disappear [6].[3] In his thinking, the nodularity observed in cases of advanced cirrhosis was simply a trapping of liver tissue rather than exuberant growth (regeneration) of liver cells.

Indeed, the liver was a peculiar organ. That nodularity observed by Ackermann was not simply a passive phenomenon from encasing connective tissue, but rather a true enlargement of liver tissue. Friedrich Theodor von Frerichs (1819–1885), pathologist at the *Charité* in Berlin, thought so. He had recognized liver hypertrophy after injury in livers gouged and scarred by syphilitic hepatitis. Uninvolved liver parenchyma swelled with plump cells that soon completely replaced loss of substance from the destructive disease [7].

And then the great German pathologist Emil Ponfick witnessed the phenomenon he called *Leber recreation*, literally, liver "recreation" by "the most powerful gland in the body." From a series of experiments in rabbits, employing techniques learned from his contemporary Themistocles Gluck, he was able to remove up to 5/6 of the lobular liver, piecemeal or all at once, without killing the animals, some even surviving beyond 24 days. "In an as yet unimagined measure, the organism shows patience with regard to even a very significant loss of liver substance," he would write in 1890 [8]. It was his observations that allowed an initial understanding of changes in the visceral circulation and abdominal organs—the mild congestion of portal blood flow yet changes that failed to disrupt important physiologic functions despite what predecessors had seen as a severe restriction of portal blood

---

[3] Ackermann makes a clear distinction between hypertrophic and atrophic cirrhosis; the former a precursor to the later and, in essence, a disease of connective tissue, a *neoplastischen* of ingrowth.

flow to the remaining liver. The liver itself seemed to maintain its role in homeostasis despite only a small fraction remaining. In later experiments, Ponfick tracked liver regrowth following subtotal removal after 2 weeks, 3 months, and, in one case, over 1 year, carefully weighing and recording liver removed at the time of surgery and at necropsy. Even by 2 weeks more than half the liver weight had been regained, an astounding burst of "glandular" activity [9]. Following "eradication," formation of young liver tissue follows that, although possessing certain peculiarities, may essentially be regarded as a substitute for the original—and begins as early as a few days after surgery, "climaxing already in a few weeks' time." This *hyperplasie* seemed to arise from preexisting cells of the lobules. Even though not a surgeon, Ponfick was convinced that surgery for liver disease would be successful without jeopardizing organ function and, particularly for the liver itself, without compromising its pivotal role, simply because of its regenerative powers. In neighboring France similar findings of regeneration were detected by the controversial surgeon Eugène-Louis Doyen (1859–1916) who found and reported in 1892 liver hypertrophy in cases of "cancer, hypertrophic cirrhosis, amyloid degeneration, and spleno-hepatic leukemia" [10].

Of course, much of the early observations of liver regeneration came from cases of fulminant liver failure, termed acute yellow atrophy. At the 55th Annual Session of the American Medical Association in Atlantic City in June 1900, William George MacCallum, resident pathologist at the new Johns Hopkins Hospital, presented the autopsy findings of a man who had died after a brief illness characterized by icterus and delirium. His liver was firm and contained distinct lobules bordered by thick connective tissue. In these lobules were enlarged liver cells with vigorous mitotic activity. There were even some bile duct cells with mitoses. MacCallum concluded that, while cirrhosis can signify significant liver destruction, numerous islets of regeneration can also be found, indicating the potential of the diseased liver to regenerate. This was termed by some as "carcinoma in cirrhosis" or "cirrhosis carcinomatosis" referring not to a true hepatocellular carcinoma but to a benign regenerative process akin to neoplasia (although it is inescapable that one should lead, at times, to the other). Of course the German pathologist Marchand had described renewal of liver cells from damaged architecture in acute yellow atrophy in 1895 in the course of his classic description of pathologic findings for this form of fulminant liver failure [11]. New liver cells arose from damaged cells, he wrote, specifying that bile duct cells did not participate in this process and their apparent proliferation were, instead, the result of renewal of parenchymal cells themselves. This would become a disputed and controversial topic. After the turn of the century pathologist Robert Muir of Glasgow might have agreed, contending that proliferation of liver cells occurred chiefly under two conditions: (1) repair following breach of continuity of structure and (2) in compensatory hypertrophy and hyperplasia. In the later condition such as exists in partial removal of liver substance, the stimulus, in his mind, seemed to result from increased metabolic activity due to some type of ill-defined molecular damage and affected only the liver cells themselves and not other components of hepatic substance such as connective tissue elements [12]. But later clinical and experimental work clearly showed that bile ducts did, indeed, participate in hepatic regeneration. In a rather extensive review of reported liver regeneration by Frederick Fishback at the Mayo Clinic in 1929, plenty of observations had been witnessed in humans following acute yellow atrophy, carcinoma, or cirrhosis, but none observed after partial liver removal. Experimentally a number of researchers had produced animal models of post-hepatectomy regeneration in rats, rabbits, and dogs.

Fundamental to understanding the process of compensatory hypertrophy a partial hepatectomy model seemed most appropriate. It most closely approximated the clinical situation following surgical extirpation of liver tissue, leaving behind hepatic parenchyma that, for the most part, was unaffected by the surgery and was otherwise healthy.[4] Such hepatocytes have enormous potential for clonal replication. Some have claimed that one individual hepatocyte could expand through a minimum of 34 cell divisions, perhaps in excess of 68, giving rise to at least 1.7×10^{10} daughter cells, enough to generate 50 rat livers [13]. It was in the rat that experimental subtotal hepatectomy was perfected.[5] With a distinct and predictable lobulated liver, partial liver resections could be performed, albeit with some practice, to provide a survivable model of liver regeneration. It was in the rat that George Higgins and Reuben Anderson, at the Mayo Clinic, showed that after 70% hepatectomy there was a burst of mitotic activity beginning on the first postoperative day. Actual division of the cells, however, did not manifest until the second day and seemed to peak by day three, corresponding to a substantial increase in liver mass that gradually tapered off by the end of the first week. A second but less pronounced growth spurt occurred around the second week, with near restoration of hepatic substance [14].

What accounted for this sudden acceleration of mitoses? Peyton Rous and Louise Larimore at the Rockefeller Institute (1917–1919) suggested that there were factors in portal blood that influenced liver cell conditioning. This was prophetically shown in their 1920 publication by ligating portal branches of the rabbit liver and observing atrophy of the involved areas [15].[6] Conversely, those parts of the liver that continued to be perfused by portal blood underwent noticeable hypertrophy as if to compensate for atrophy of affected parts. Similarly, Dutch physician-scientist Leendert Schalm and his colleagues in Utrecht, Netherlands, in 1952 had observed little change in bilirubin metabolism in patients whose livers were massively replaced with tumor, obstructing many of the bile ducts. They proceeded to show compensatory hypertrophy in pig and rabbit livers with ligation of biliary ducts to the majority of liver lobes. The ligated lobes became atrophic while there was

---

[4] Of course, the alternate model was widespread hepatocyte destruction using some form of cytotoxic agent. The concern was that the agent might have affected all populations of hepatocytes, even viable ones, which might impair their ability to regenerate.

[5] "Compensatory hypertrophy" rather than regeneration is, strictly speaking, a more accurate term. The post-hepatectomy liver does not actually "grow" the resected lobe, but rather diffusely enlarges to match the pre-resection mass.

[6] A graduate of Johns Hopkins School of Medicine, devoted much of his career to virology, winning the Nobel Prize in Physiology or Medicine in 1966 for his work in tumor-inducing viruses.

enlargement of remaining lobes so that the total mass of liver remained essentially unchanged [16]. Their work determined that both bile duct occlusion and portal vein occlusion stimulated hypertrophy in remaining liver and atrophy in the affected parts, maintaining liver cell mass and hepatocyte function. What was the stimulus? Was this a local phenomenon or systemic? Were there indeed splanchnic factors at play?

A major setback to this theory occurred when New York surgeon Charles Child and his team showed no slowing of regeneration of dog liver when portocaval transposition diverted splanchnic blood into the systemic circulation and systemic blood into the liver. "Portal blood itself is not essential for liver regeneration ... failure of liver regeneration ... is due to diminished hepatic blood flow," they wrote in 1953 [17]. This notion persisted for another dozen years until Starzl's group in Denver convincingly showed in 1965 that canine auxiliary liver transplants thrived with splanchnic blood while native livers, now deprived of portal blood, withered [18]. Further experiments in split transposition of portal flow showed similar results. Portal flow maintained "health" of the perfused liver segments [19]. Similar findings were reported in a series of three patients, all of whom died after auxiliary liver transplantation in which the allograft was, for the most part, deprived of portal blood flow. Each of the necropsies displayed evidence of liver transplant atrophy much more severe than seen in any orthotopic allograft. Splanchnic flow, and a good deal of it, seemed necessary just for maintenance of normal architecture and morphology [20]. An important study by Frederick Moolten and Nancy Bucher at Harvard University in 1967 exposed a vital humoral factor contained in the systemic circulation of hepatectomized rats that induced incorporation of radio-labeled thymidine into hepatic DNA of resting rats by carotid-to-jugular cross-circulation [21]. By 1975 using ingenious split flow experiments in dogs, shunting pancreatic blood to one side of the liver and splanchnic visceral flow to the other, Starzl's group had demonstrated insulin to be a dominant humoral factor in hepatic regeneration. Other splanchnic agents were suspect as well [22].

Perhaps no one investigator has been more instrumental in understanding hepatic regeneration, though, than Harvard Professor Nancy Bucher (1913–2017). Doctor Bucher's career was meteoric. She attended Bryn Mawr College in Pennsylvania and then enrolled in medical school at the Johns Hopkins University. She was the first woman to receive a medical degree from the Johns Hopkins School of Medicine, graduating in 1943. As a burgeoning young pathologist she joined the Huntington Laboratory at the Massachusetts General Hospital and the faculty of Harvard Medical School. Her chief and mentor Joseph Aub encouraged her to investigate cancer cell growth and introduced her to Higgins' model of rat partial hepatectomy in 1946. Her first publication on regeneration appeared in 1950 in Cancer Research on the effect of age (rat) on hepatic regeneration, documenting by histologic nuclear assessment, that age between adult and senile rats did not dramatically affect the rate of regrowth [23]. Her inaugural exposure to circulating humoral substances initiating regeneration was reported 1 year later, in 1951, with an ingenious experimental model for cross-circulation called parabiosis, in which skin and subcutaneous tissue from littermate rats were sutured together, thus promoting cross-circulation and sharing of systemic agents. In this experiment one of the parabiotic pairs was hepatectomized that resulted in accelerated mitoses in the normal rat, thus establishing a systemic stimulus, rather than simply a local, liver-based reaction, to regeneration [24]. The curiosity about liver hyperplasia and hypertrophy was that, as opposed to other tissue like bone marrow, liver regeneration does not require the presence of stem cells as a prerequisite. Regeneration takes place by redirection of existing mature hepatocytes and other populations of cells in the remnant organ.

By 1963, Bucher had compiled an impressive array of research data concerning hepatic regeneration following partial hepatectomy in the rat model. She described the morphological sequence of events immediately following extirpation affecting, primarily, parenchymal hepatocytes resulting within 24 h by onset of mitoses. Initiators of such an elaborate synthetic process remained a mystery, however, and formed the basis for her continued research in this area. In terms of regenerative control, she suggested four possible mechanisms: (1) overloading of the excretory function; (2) a shift in blood flow; (3) a fall in lipid peroxides; or (4) a change in composition of the blood. However, to sort out these options was simply beyond the availability of sound research data [25].

Bucher concurred with Starzl that hormonal factors insulin and glucagon are indeed involved in regeneration, working synergistically with epidermal growth factor (EGF) [26]. She, however, could not verify by experimentation in rats that either glucagon or insulin were prime triggers for mitosis. Eviscerated rats undergoing partial hepatectomy still were able to mount a regenerative response without portal blood flow, although the regenerative capability was substantially enhanced by the synergistic combination of insulin and glucagon. Bucher thus implied a dual stimulus to regeneration (hyperplasia and hypertrophy) by systemic and splanchnic agents. "[A] critical factor in hepatic regeneration is the synergistic action of both pancreatic hormones, which in combination give major impetus to the growth process," she commented [27].

In a follow-up article in 1991 Nancy Bucher summarized the state of knowledge in regeneration, citing hormones (including glucagon, insulin, and prostaglandins), growth factor—particularly hepatocyte growth factor—and cell-cell and cell-matrix local interactions. Her lifelong work in the field and overall comprehension of the epistemology of regeneration added insight and direction to any number of future investigations [28]. At about that time George Michalopoulos moved to the University of Pittsburgh Medical Center as Chair of the Department of Pathology. His research focused on initiators and terminators of liver regeneration in the partial hepatectomy model. "Few aspects of liver regeneration have spawned as much research as the quest to find what triggers the regenerative response," he and colleague Marie DeFrances wrote in 1997. In all the phenotypic changes that occur with mitogenesis, hepatocytes still provide differentiated cellular functions such as glucose regulation, synthesis, secretion of bile, and detoxification, prompting Michalopoulos and DeFrances to term them the "phenotypic acrobat" [1].

Research since has focused on three main areas of compensatory hypertrophy in partial hepatectomy models: the initiation or priming phase; the proliferation phase;

and the termination phase. Immediately after partial hepatectomy the remnant liver is suddenly exposed to greater portal blood flow and multiples of the normal concentration of systemic and splanchnic signaling factors. While this seems intuitively central to the regenerative process, evidence has not conclusively demonstrated the exact role, only that diversion of portal flow after hepatectomy diminishes regeneration, and too great portal flow and/or portal pressure can be damaging to hepatocytes and detrimental to regeneration. And what stops it? Again, research has not yet provided definitive answers, but it is likely a combination of key metabolites, growth factors, cytokines, and, importantly, restoration of some type of three-dimensional matrix may provide an aggregate of signals terminating the process. "For practical purposes," Michalopoulos said in 2014, "we should consider that there is a complex process composed of many signals that functions as a 'hepatostat', adjusting the size of the liver to the needs of the body" [29]. Indeed, in this whirlwind activity there seems to be a manifestation of Plato's appetitive soul.

Does the presence of cirrhosis impair regenerative capabilities of the human liver? In 1965, TY Lin in Taipei demonstrated depressed regenerative capabilities of the cirrhotic liver compared to non-cirrhotic livers undergoing partial hepatectomy (right or left "lobectomy") as measured by serial enlargement of remnant livers marked with radiopaque clips. Non-cirrhotic livers showed restoration of liver mass in 4 to 13 months after resection; not so in cirrhotic livers. In fact, in cirrhotic livers, despite slight enlargement at 3 weeks, there was no appreciable enlargement thereafter (up to 1 year later) [30]. Even microscopically, evidence of "new" regeneration, outside preoperative regenerative nodules typical of cirrhotic livers, was not detected in Lin's follow-up clinical study. "[A] cirrhotic liver remnant never shows a postoperative increase in size even after one year," he commented. In contrast, in non-cirrhotic liver remnants a true regenerative hyperplasia occurred which, in Lin's estimation, contributed to restoration of normal liver function. There seemed to be a lag phase of 3 to 7 days post-resection before any increase in size could be appreciated by ^{99m}technicium liver scanning [31].

How has this impacted clinical liver surgery? Perhaps one could "grow" liver tissue, not in the laboratory, in vitro, but in an actual patient in preparation for extirpative surgery. Clearly, advances in surgical technique, anatomic understanding, and anesthesia had permitted resection of large volumes of liver. The major danger was no longer fatal hemorrhage but simply the size of the remnant liver. Would it be sizeable enough to sustain metabolic function and life itself? Even with that, would it be suffient to initiate and sustain regeneration? A critical mass of liver was necessary for this to occur. With split-liver transplantation, reduced-sized allografts (particularly left lateral sectors into adults) had sometimes been too small to fulfill metabolic functions and allow regeneration. "Small-for-size" remnant was the term applied. Similarly, following resection small remnants failed to function or regenerate as if there was a critical volume below which hepatocytes were incapable of acting.

Why was this? It seemed more to do with blood flow than mass itself. Volumes and patterns of portal blood bathing remaining liver cells could affect the delicate, interplay of liver cell, sinusoidal cell, and Kupffer cell, unbalancing basic excretory, synthetic, and detoxifying functions and transmission of signals and initiators for regeneration.[7] It indeed was a flow problem, not necessarily a volume problem.

By the late 1990s, Japanese surgeon Masatoshi Makuuchi had developed an expansive program in hepatobiliary surgery at the University of Tokyo. Between 1990 and 1993 he had already performed 16 living donor liver transplants (deceased donors were a rarity in Asia). While the donor liver portions were smaller than ideal liver mass, there was no instance of postoperative liver failure, and each graft increased rapidly in size [34].[8] Extrapolating from his transplant experience, Makuuchi's team began using CT prospectively to determine adequacy of the future liver remnant, finding that patients with normal livers could reliably undergo up to resection of 60% of their liver mass [36]. Most clinicians now agreed that minimum future liver remnant should be in excess of 25% of the total liver volume, and for diseased livers above 40%.[9] For minimum transplant allograft size Makuuchi's Japanese team suggested a graft to recipient body weight ratio exceeding 0.8% [34].

In vivo liver growth after transplantation and the importance of portal blood had captured Makuuchi's interest. The observations of Cantlie, Rous, and Schalm had not gone unnoticed. Sectoral deprivation of portal flow could be advantageous in enhancing growth of the remaining perfused liver. Even prior to his transplant work, in 1990, Makuuchi, noting that patients with hilar cholangiocarcinoma and an obstructed right portal vein did better following extended lobectomies, incorporated radiographic occlusion of the right portal vein into his preoperative preparation. Portal vein embolization was done by occlusion with a gelatin powder mixture of the involved branch of the portal vein either intraoperatively by accessing the ileo-colic vein or percutaneously accessing the right hepatic vein and puncturing through into the portal system. After a mean interval of 17 days the operation was performed.[10] A modest but noticeable increase in size of the future liver remnant was detected. Extended right or left hepatic resections were performed to incorporate all tumor-bearing tissue. Of 14 subjects there was only one postoperative death, testifying to the effectiveness of this therapy to promote, almost like a "head-start," the regenerative process. These encouraging results from Japan led to widespread use of portal vein embolization to stimulate preoperative enlargement and augmentation

---

[7] All is still largely speculation and not the purpose of this work to investigate. For a summary see Refs. [32] and [33].

[8] His group had reported their first case of an adult recipient of a left liver graft in 1994. This liver quickly enlarged to a volume of 1141 mL within 2 weeks of the transplant [35].

[9] An early study supported the use of CT (computerized tomography) in measuring liver volume employing explanted livers for transplant for verification. See Ref. [37].

[10] Makuuchi actually had reported his initial results in the Japanese literature in 1984. His first case was done 2 years before, in 1982 [38]. Kenichi Takayusu published a follow-up report on the observation that patients with tumor occlusion of branches of the portal vein had atrophic ipsilateral lobes while there was compensatory hypertrophy of the contralateral lobes [39]. This prompted further study with intentional occlusion. Of course regeneration in experimental animals takes longer, up to 6 weeks. However, in Makuuchi's series the concern was tumor progression to unresectability. Therefore surgery was carried out with a shorter interval. See the original published article: [40].

of the future liver remnant. Teleologically, the remnant hepatocytes, now "seeing" enhanced portal blood flow and higher concentrations of signalers, initiators, and promoters of regeneration acts as if neighboring liver has either been destroyed or removed and acts accordingly. The practice quickly gained popularity in efforts to adequately address primary hepatocellular carcinoma and metastatic colorectal disease, producing a population of patients previously not thought suitable for resection because of small residual liver mass.[11] Effectiveness was eventually demonstrated statistically by a meta-analysis study of 37 clinical trials published in 2008 that showed percutaneous transhepatic portal embolization produced a mean increase in remnant liver volume of almost 12% [42]. However, the period of regenerative hyperplasia could take not less than four and as long as 8 weeks before the future liver remnant was of sufficient size.

And for those patients where the delay required by standard portal vein embolization would threaten to allow growth of targeted cancerous lesions, surgeons at the Bavarian University of Regensburg developed a two-stage operation designed to enhance compensatory regeneration. The method was uncovered quite by happenstance. One of the surgeons had backed out of a formidable extended right hepatectomy for hilar cholangiocarcinoma—he felt the future liver remnant was simply too small to sustain life—but had already divided liver parenchyma through Segment IV. He performed a bile duct anastomosis to the lateral segments and ligated the portal vein. By chance a CT scan some days later demonstrated a dramatic enlargement of his lateral segments, as if the act of parenchymal division and portal vein ligation had provided an extra stimulus for reactive hyperplasia. So the process was purposely repeated in other patients with similar lesions. Ligation of portal vein and splitting of the liver along anatomic right and left planes (while keeping venous drainage intact), fully stripping the watershed area of Segment IV, in fact allowed for much more rapid hyperplasia and regeneration of the future liver remnant. Results were impressive. The second stage of the operation could be done not weeks in the future but an average of *9 days* later. Complete devascularization seemed central to the accelerated regenerative process, a task not easy to accomplish radiographically. It is as if the diseased and excluded right liver could still act as an auxiliary liver to assist the remnant liver during those crucial days before hyperplasia was in full swing.

Before long the Germans had collected 25 such cases. As lead investigator, Andreas Schnitzbauer from Regensburg reported an amazing 74% volume increase in the future liver remnant those several days before the second-stage hepatectomy. No patient developed irreversible liver failure following surgery [43]. The new strategy was eventually termed "Associating Liver Partition and Portal Vein Ligation for Staged Hepatectomy," or ALPPS for short. By 2014, 202 patients with complete data sets from 99 centers were gathered for the International ALPPS Registry. Just as in the early Regensburg experience, this radical partitioning strategy resulted in a

---

[11]The Paris group at the *Hôpital Paul Brousse* headed efforts to utilize this technique, which was soon championed by legendary liver surgeon Henri Bismuth. See Ref. [41].

mean enlargement of the future liver remnant of 80% [44]. "This technique read-dresses the current management of locally advanced liver malignancies and opens a new chapter in the history of liver surgery," so wrote Eduardo de Santibañes from Buenos Aires and Pierre Clavien from Zurich in an editorial commentary on ALPPS [45]. It seemed as if this anatomic and physiologic manipulation maximized innate capabilities of the mammalian liver to regenerate, as if Prometheus, unchained from his perch in the Caucasus, had descended to bestow on mortals below his lessons of restoration.

References

1. Michalopoulos GK, DeFrances MC (1997) Liver regeneration. Science 276:60–66
2. Grote G (1865) Plato, and the other companions of Sokrates. John Murray, London, p 287
3. Coxe JR (1846) Writings of Hippocrates and Galen. Lindsay and Blakiston, Philadelphia
4. Liddell HG, Scott R (1871) A lexicon abridged from Liddell and Scott's Greek-English lexicon. Clarendon Press, Oxford
5. Cruveilhier J (1845) *Traite d'Anatomie Descriptive,* Tome Troisieme. Maison Bechet Jeune, Paris, p 387
6. Ackermann T (1880) Ueber hypertrophische und atrophische Lebercirrhose. Archiv für pathologische Anatomie und Physiologie und für klinische Medicin 80:396–436
7. Frerichs F (1861) Klinik der Leberkrankheiten, Bd II. Braunschweig, Friedrich Vieweg und Sohn, p 203
8. Ponfick E (1890) Ueber die Folgen einer theilweisen Entfernung der Leber. Jahres-Bericht der Schlesischen Gesellschaft:38–39
9. Ponfick E (1890) Experimentelle Beiträge zur Pathologie der Leber. Archiv für pathologische Anatomie und Physiologie 119:193–240
10. Doyen E (1892) Quelques Operations sur le Foie et les Voies Biliares. Archives Provinciales de Chirurgie 1:149–178
11. Marchand F (1895) Ueber Ausgang der Acuten Leberatrophie im Multiple Knotige Hyperplasia. Beitr z path Anat u z allg Path 17:206–219
12. Muir R (1907) On proliferation of the cells of the liver. J Pathol 12:287–305
13. Overturf K, Al-Dhalimy M, Ou C-N, Grompe M (1997) Serial transplantation reveals the stem-cell-like regenerative potential of adult mouse hepatocytes. Am J Pathol 151:1273–1280
14. Higgins GM (1931) Experimental pathology of the liver: I. restoration of the liver of the white rat following partial surgical removal. Arch Pathol 12:186–202
15. Rous PL (1920) Relation of the portal blood to liver maintenance: a demonstration of liver atrophy conditional on compensation. J Exp Med 31:609–632
16. Schalm LS et al (1952) The regenerative power of the liver and its reserve capacity for excreting bile. Lancet 259:75–81
17. Child CI (1953) Liver regeneration following portocaval transposition in dogs. Ann Surg 138:600–608
18. Marchioro TP et al (1965) Physiologic requirements for auxiliary liver homotransplantation. Surg Gynecol Obstet 121:17–31
19. Marchioro TP et al (1967) The effect of partial portacaval transposition on the canine liver. Surgery 61:723–732
20. Halgrimson CG et al (1966) Auxiliary liver transplantation: effect of host portocaval shunt: experimental and clinical observations. Arch Surg 93:107–118
21. Moolten FL, Bucher NLR (1967) Regeneration of rat liver: transfer of humoral agent by cross circulation. Science 158:272–274

22. Starzl TE, Porter KA, Kashiwagi N (1975) Portal hepatotrophic factors, diabetes mellitus and acute liver atrophy, hypertrophy and regeneration. Surg Gynecol Obstet 141:843–858

23. Bucher NL, Glinos AD (1950) The effect of age on regeneration of rat liver. Cancer Res 10:324–332

24. Bucher NL, Scott JF, Aub JC (1951) Regeneration of the liver in parabiotic rats. Cancer Res 11:457–465

25. Bucher NL (1963) Regeneration of mammalian liver. Int Rev Cytol 15:245–300

26. Bucher NL, Patel U, Cohen S (1977) Hormonal factors concerned with liver regeneration. Ciba Found Symp 55:95–107

27. Bucher NL, Swaffield MN (1976) Synergistic action of insulin and glucagon in hepatic regeneration. Lancet 1:646

28. Bucher NL (1991) Liver regeneration: an overview. J Gastroenterol Hepatol 6:615–624

29. Michalopoulos GK (2014) Advances in liver regeneration. Ex Rev Gastroenterol Hepatol 8:897–907

30. Lin T-Y, Chen C-C (1965) Metabolic function and regeneration of cirrhotic and non-cirrhotic livers after hepatic lobectomy in man. Ann Surg 162:959–972

31. Lin T-Y, Lee C-S, Chen C-C et al (1979) Regeneration of human liver after hepatic lobectomy studied by repeated liver scanning and repeated needle biopsy. Ann Surg 190:48–53

32. Golritz M, Majlesara A, Sakka SE et al (2016) Small for size and flow (SFSF) syndrome: an alternative description for posthepatectomy liver failure. Clin Res Hepatol Gastroenterol 40:267–275

33. Tucker ON, Heaton N (2005) The 'small for size' liver syndrome. Curr Opin Crit Care 11:150–155

34. Kawasaki SM et al (1998) Living related liver transplantation in adults. Ann Surg 227:269–274

35. Hashikura YM et al (1994) Successful living-related partial liver transplantation to an adult patient. Lancet 343:1233–1234

36. Kubota KM et al (1997) Measurement of liver volume and hepatic functional reserve as a guide to decision-making in Resectional surgery for hepatic tumors. Hepatology 26:1176–1181

37. Van Thiel DH et al (1985) In vivo hepatic volume determination using sonography and computed tomography. Gastroenterology 88:1812–1817

38. Makuuchi MT et al (1984) Preoperative transcatheter embolization of the portal venous branch for patients receiving extended lobectomy due to the bile duct carcinoma. J Jpn Surg Assoc 45:1558–1564

39. Takayusu KM et al (1986) Hepatic lobar atrophy following obstruction of the ipsilateral portal vein from hilar cholangiocarcinoma. Radiology 160:389–393

40. Makuuchi MT et al (1990) Preoperative portal embolization to increase safety of major hepatectomy for hilar bile duct carcinoma: a preliminary report. Surgery 107:521–527

41. Azoulay DC et al (2000) Resection of nonresectable liver metastases from colorectal cancer after percutaneous portal vein embolization. Ann Surg 231:480–486

42. Abulkhir AL et al (2008) Preoperative portal vein embolization for major liver resection. Ann Surg 247:49–57

43. Schnitzbauer AA et al (2012) Right portal vein ligation combined with in situ splitting induces rapid left lateral liver lobe hypertrophy enabling 2-staged extended right hepatic resection in small-for-size settings. Ann Surg 255:405–414

44. Schadde EA-C et al (2014) Early survival and safety of ALPPS: first report of the international ALPPS registry. Ann Surg 260:829–838

45. Santibañes EC-A et al (2012) Playing play-Doh to prevent postoperative liver failure: the "ALPPS" approach. Ann Surg 255:415–417

Chapter 15
Prometheus Renewed

An enormous number of liver resections have now been performed, tens of thousands. According to the United States National Inpatient Sample from 2000 to 2012 31,084 open liver resection were recorded with operative mortality generally below 6% [1].[1] With published studies worldwide of resection for colorectal metastases over the 30 year period from 1987 to 2016 alone, 5207 patients were tabulated for one meta-analysis [2]. Thousands of patients have undergone resections using minimally invasive surgery but adhering to principles no less relevant than open operations: exposure, mobilization, inflow control, and hemostatic parenchymal separation [3]. In less than half a century Jean Lortat-Jacob's bold adventure in Paris has now become almost commonplace practice in many medical centers. And the pessimistic opinion concerning the much maligned total liver transplant was turned on its ear by daunting efforts of pioneers across the globe that have laid fertile ground for numbers of second and third generation transplanters to give new futures to what were considered hopeless cases decades ago. And this is but a snapshot. Work has not halted. Patients still flock for the relief of metastatic malignancies or burgeoning hepatic cancers. Sallow-eyed, wasted victims of cirrhosis wait patiently for their turn at a second life. The lines will never shorten. It will be the tireless efforts of surgeon-scientists to expand the pathways for correction of nature's miscalculations. Through rigorous experimentation and plodding determinism these intense individuals will follow in the footsteps of Lortat-Jacob and Hepp and Starzl. As Harvey Cushing stressed, over a century ago:

> The real leaders of to-day in surgery owe their place not to any special brilliance in operative manipulation, but to their laborious experimental investigations of certain problems of disease, whereby has been disclosed a rational mechanical basis for surgical therapy which can then be safely and successfully adapted by their many followers [4].

---

[1] Remember the National Inpatient Sample is simply that—a sample of hospitals. The true numbers are not known but very likely multiples of that.

© The Editor(s) (if applicable) and The Author(s), under exclusive license to
Springer Nature Switzerland AG 2020
T. S. Helling, D. Azoulay, *Historical Foundations of Liver Surgery*,
https://doi.org/10.1007/978-3-030-47095-1_15

The liver is unique among visceral organs, tying together the machinery of ingestion, digestion, and excretion, processing the many substances so essential for survival. Understanding of its inner workings and metabolic pathways has given physicians the opportunity to rearrange and manipulate for the acquired conditions that can affect this vital structure. And it has been surgeons who have led the crusade to unravel its mysteries and conquer the formidable responses to injury that held off so many *ancien* physicians. And into the future it will continue to be surgeons who will take discoveries of the laboratories and apply them directly to the human frame, to augment, hamper, or eradicate nature's basic tendencies.

Future frontiers in neoplastic liver disease rests more likely on refining blood-borne agents, immunotherapy, and directed ionizing radiation (if not newer, as yet undiscovered, energy sources) than on any further efforts to extirpate tumors. The principles of safe and oncologically sound liver surgery have been well worked out by the legions of surgical pioneers discussed in this text. Surgery will be but one weapon in the practitioner's armamentarium to address the lethality and metastatic potential of cancers.

As for chronic liver disease and the need for liver replacement, continued efforts to blunt the body's immunologic defenses for specific acceptance (tolerance) of foreign antigens will be key to long-term survival. Limiting factors of donor availability have done much to confine access to new livers and will continue to be a challenge into the future. Use of partitioned livers, while applicable in the pediatric age groups still has serious limitations in the adult recipient population. Perhaps new agents will be found to catalyze and accelerate regeneration, affording the host benefits of heretofore considered small-for-size allografts. However, the very fact that livers can be exchanged between humans in a safe and functional manner is the cornerstone to this particular therapy, unheard of just decades ago. The brave procession of early recipients and the resolute and skill of their stalwart surgeons is testimony to the ever-hopeful and inquisitive human spirit.

This, then, is the seemingly eternal cycle of human endeavor, striving to undue or alter the basic flaws in mortal existence: those scientist-pioneers always curious, always inquisitive, until excellence itself is within grasp. And then, without hesitation, resuming the pursuit—even though certainly unattainable—of immortality itself. As Ernest Lewis said over a century ago to his fellow surgeons of the *Southern Surgical and Gynecological Association*:

> With a more profound appreciation of the subtle factors of surgical diseases and a deeper knowledge of their pathology we may in time attain the perfection of surgical science and effect cures in cases now relegated to the knife, and which stand in evidence of the surgeon's impotency or incompetency [5].

And perfection can only come at the expense of intense devotion and study. So it is now that the realm of liver surgery has become a specialty of its own. And deservedly so. To once again quote the great Harvey Cushing:

> [G]ranting the wisdom and necessity of a general surgical training beforehand, I do not see how such particularization of work can be avoided, if we wish more surely and progressively to advance our manipulative therapy [4].

The character of these new pioneers will be rich with enthusiasm, hope, and compassion. Who would have thought that from those tentative efforts to staunch dark bleeding from liver trauma would spring surgeons capable of replacing the whole thing? More miracles—but not miracles at all, really—await the pioneering efforts of future Starzls and Bismuths and Makuuchis through the tiniest of steps, the smallest of successes, the greatest of disappointments, and the ever-present desire to walk back in that laboratory or that operating room, change it up, and try it again. Such is the human spirit. Such is the march of determination.

References

1. He JA, Amini N, Spolverato G et al (2015) National trends with a laparoscopic liver resection: results from a population-based analysis. HPB 17:919–926
2. Tang HB et al (2016) Comparison of anatomical and nonanatomical hepatectomy for colorectal liver metastasis: a meta-analysis of 5207 patients. Sci Rep 6:32,304. https://doi.org/10.1038/srep32304
3. Reddy SK et al (2011) Laparoscopic liver resection. World J Surg 35:1478–1486
4. Cushing H (1905) The special field of neurological surgery. Bull Johns Hopkins Hosp 16:77–87
5. Lewis ES (1897) The President's address. Trans Southern Surg Gynecol Assoc 9:1–8

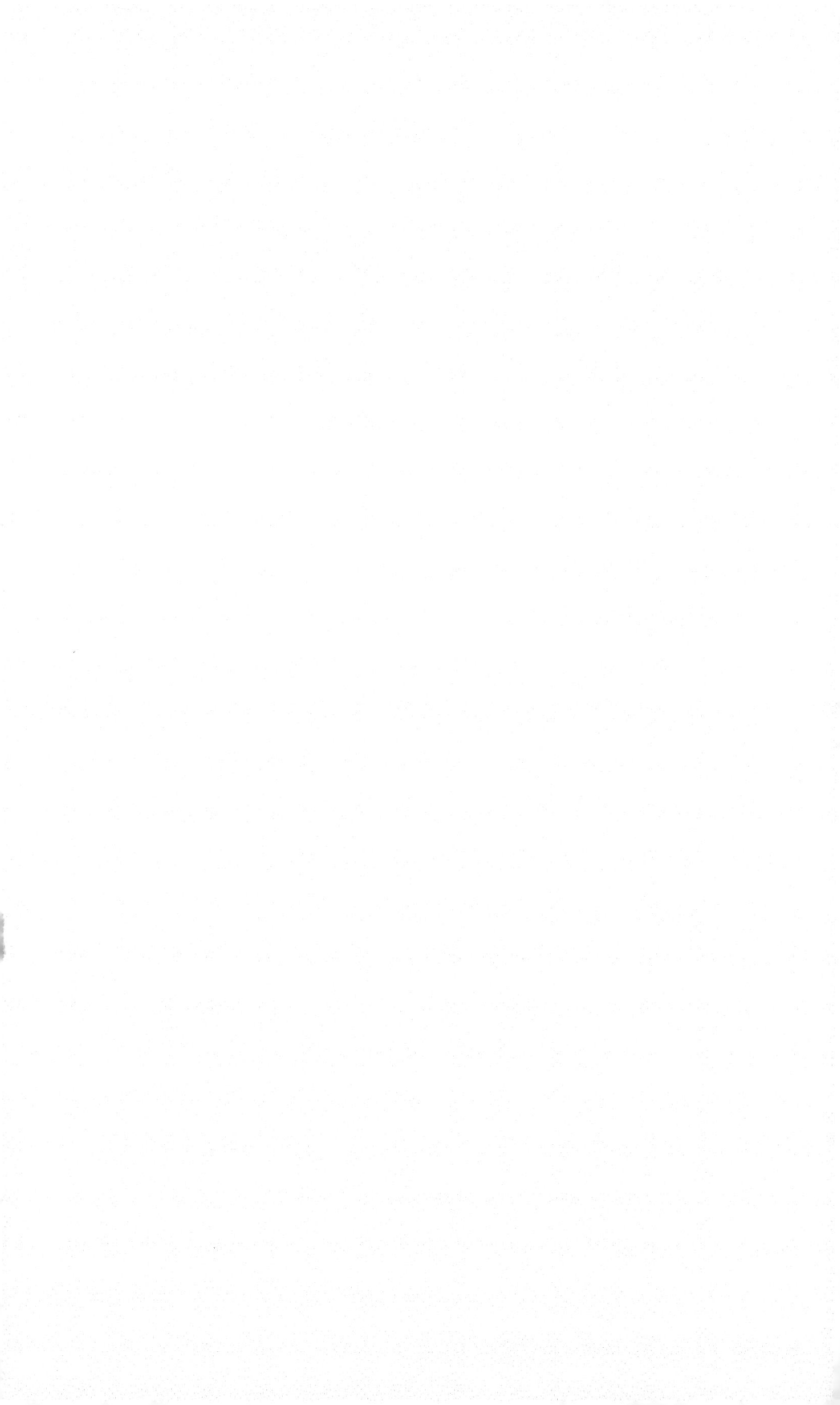

The manufacturer's authorised representative in the EU is Springer
Nature Customer Service Centre GmbH, Europaplatz 3, 69115 Heidelberg,
Germany. If you have any concerns regarding our products, please
contact ProductSafety@springernature.com

Printed and bound by CPI Group (UK) Ltd, Croydon, CR0 4YY

29/04/2026

02099519-0003